# Fitness Facts

## The Healthy Living Handbook

**B. Don Franks, PhD**
Louisiana State University

**Edward T. Howley, PhD**
University of Tennessee

*Human Kinetics Books*
Champaign, Illinois

## Dedication

Alice and Ray Franks
Sean, Chris, and Geoffrey Howley

**Library of Congress Cataloging-in-Publication Data**

Franks, B. Don.
    Fitness facts : the healthy living handbook / B. Don Franks,
Edward T. Howley.
      p.    cm.
    Bibliography: p.
    Includes index.
    ISBN 0-87322-229-6
    1. Physical fitness.  I. Howley, Edward T., 1943-    . II. Title.
GV481.F725  1989
613.7'1--dc19                  88-37133
                                    CIP

ISBN: 0-87322-229-6

Developmental Editor: Marie Roy
Copyeditor: Barbara Walsh
Assistant Editors: Holly Gilly and Valerie Hall
Proofreader: Linda Siegel
Production Director: Ernie Noa
Typesetter: Sandra Meier
Text Design: Keith Blomberg
Text Layout: Denise Peters
Cover Design: Jack Davis
Cover Photo: Wilmer Zehr
Illustrations: George Moudry, EdD, and Valerie Hall
Symbols: Susan Metros, PhD
Printer: United Graphics
*Special thanks to Terri Wetzel, Tim Patrick, Laurie Ellsworth, and Scott Stevenson.*

Printed in the United States of America

10  9  8  7  6  5  4  3  2

**Human Kinetics Books**
A Division of Human Kinetics Publishers, Inc.
Box 5076, Champaign, IL 61825-5076
1-800-747-4HKP

*UK Office:*
Human Kinetics Publishers (UK) Ltd.
P.O. Box 18
Rawdon, Leeds LS19 6TG
England
(0532) 504211

# Contents

We wrote *Fitness Facts* to share with you the fun, the benefits, and the necessary cautions of physical activity. If even a few readers experience better health and quality of life by participating safely in enjoyable activities, our effort will have been well spent.

# Acknowledgments

We want to thank Wendy Bubb, Sue Carver, Brenda Copeland, Mark Hector, Jean Lewis, Wendell Liemohn, Daniel Martin, Barbara Porter, and Gina Sharpe. Their contributions to the *Health/Fitness Instructor's Handbook* (1986) were invaluable to us as we developed this book.

Thanks to Neil Sol and Thomas Collinwood for helpful suggestions on an earlier draft. We appreciate authors and publishers who were kind enough to allow us to use materials from their articles and books. We are indebted to our former professors, our students, and professional colleagues in AAHPERD and ACSM, too numerous to list, who have educated us over the past three decades.

Finally, thanks to the folks at Human Kinetics. Rainer Martens, Julie Simon, and our developmental editor, Marie Roy, have provided encouragement and assistance in numerous ways.

# Key to Symbols

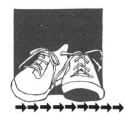

**Look ahead.**  Indicates topics to be covered in chapter.

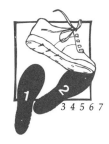

**Important point.**  Indicates a section of the discussion that should be emphasized.

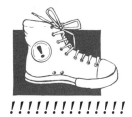

**Steps.**  Indicates a sequence or procedure.

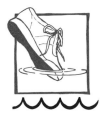

**Caution.**  Indicates a section on safety precautions.

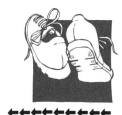

**Look back.**  Indicates the summary section.

# WHAT IS THE FIT AND HEALTHY LIFE?

**How Is the Fit and Healthy Life Defined?**
**How Is Health and Fitness Status Evaluated?**
**Where Should I Start?**

It is appropriate to begin *Fitness Facts* with concepts of fitness, health, and performance. Our society's increased emphasis on and interest in a healthy lifestyle have resulted in some confusion, as many different persons and groups promote their own particular aspects of health, fitness, and performance.

Chapter 1 deals with the definition of fitness and its relationship to health, everyday life, and performance. Chapter 2 provides procedures to determine your fitness level, and chapter 3 suggests the type of program or referral appropriate for you based on your current health status.

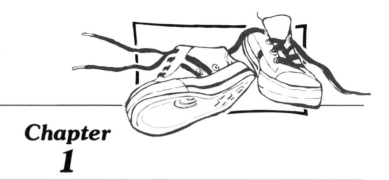

## Chapter
## 1

# Why Bother?

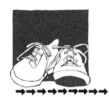

→→→→→→→→→

> **What Is Fitness?**
> **How Is Fitness Related to Health?**
> **What Are My Risks of Developing Health Problems?**
> **What Are My Fitness Goals?**
> **How Can I Gain Control Over My Health?**

In the most basic sense, you have no option but to deal with fitness and health. The only question is whether you will approach them directly and intelligently, be persuaded by the best advertising, or simply let your fitness and health be determined by default by allowing decisions in other parts of your life to determine your health status.

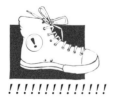

!!!!!!!!!!!!!!!

**A number of tables are provided to assist your fitness assessment. We strongly encourage you to complete these forms honestly and as completely as possible. You can submit these charts to the fitness leader if you are in a fitness program, or you can use the information for self-evaluation.**

Determining your level of satisfaction (Table 1.1) with and things that bother you (Table 1.2) about your current fitness level will provide a start for deciding what areas of your life you should consider changing.

This book provides the information you need to set up your own fitness program. Or you may decide to work with health and fitness professionals to assist you in making healthy changes in your life. In either case, *you* have to decide what changes you want to make. The old joke, "How many psychologists does it take to change a light bulb? Only one, but it has to really want to change!" applies to fitness changes as well. Tables 1.1 and 1.2 identify areas of your life that bother you or that you think need some attention. These get through the daily routine can provide the base for starting a fitness program to achieve a higher level of positive health and reduce your risk of health problems. Those interested in performing high levels of sport or other physical skills can build upon the fitness base by concentrating on ways to improve the specific performance.

The first level of health and fitness is the medical diagnosis that we are *free from disease* (a condition the medical establishment unfortunately refers to as "apparently healthy"). This is the minimum goal for all of us. We try to prevent sickness, illness, and known diseases. This is an important first step, but as terms such as "positive health" and "wellness" attempt to communicate, there is much more to health than being without disease.

The second layer deals with the *ability to carry out typical activities* at work, at home, and in leisure pursuits *without undue fatigue*. The characteristics necessary for this level differ depending on your vocation and lifestyle and differ from those of other people. The emphasis here is not on how well you perform the physical tasks, but rather that you can do them comfortably with energy left over for other things. This ensures that you have enough energy to engage in fitness activities to enhance your health and fitness status.

The final layer includes individuals who have achieved a high level of fitness and now choose to participate in certain activities. The *performance* element involves developing those skills and underlying abilities needed to do the activity well enough to compete with others (or self) at a desired level. The activities and desired level will, of course, vary among individuals. You may want to play in the "A" division of the adult soccer league or simply to play well in a pickup game of basketball on the weekend. The underlying performance abilities (e.g., agility, coordination, power, speed) and the specific sports skills will, of course, vary depending on the desired activity.

## What Is Health-Related Fitness?

Mental, emotional, and physical health serve as a base for everyone's total fitness. The family, public education, and other institutions in our society provide us with experiences that promote a healthy life. Regular exercise, a healthy diet, living without substance abuse, and coping with stressors can positively influence many of the primary and secondary risks to health. In addition to helping prevent health problems, these behaviors are the basis for a higher quality of life.

One prerequisite for becoming fit is to understand the characteristics and behaviors that are related to positive and negative health. The risks determined from epidemiological studies of large populations are normally divided into primary and secondary risk factors. *Primary* risk factors are characteristics that are strongly associated with a particular health problem independent of all other variables. For example, if you smoke (a primary risk factor), you have a high risk of heart disease even if no other risk factors are present. *Secondary* risk factors, on the other hand, have a high relationship with the health problem only when other factors are present. For example, if one of your parents died at an early age from heart disease (a secondary risk factor), you are at increased risk only if other risk factors are present. Another way to classify risk factors is to distinguish inherited risk factors that cannot be altered from lifestyle behaviors that can be modified.

### What Risks Are Unavoidable?

Some risk factors are easily identified but unfortunately can't be altered. The following segments of the population have a greater risk of heart disease, especially if they adopt unhealthy behaviors:

- Those with a family history of the disease
- Older people
- Men
- Blacks

It is important to point out that these are secondary risk factors for heart disease. They cause you to be at high risk only when added to other risk factors. In addition, part of the risk associated with family history and age are behaviors that can be changed. Family history risks include unhealthy dietary, activity, smoking, and stress behaviors that tend to be transmitted from parents to children. These types of behaviors can be corrected with proper attention throughout life, especially in early childhood. In terms of aging, it has been shown that many fitness characteristics (e.g., cardiovascular function, percent body fat) deteriorate with each passing decade. This decline, which starts in the middle 20s, has been called the "aging curve." However, the decline in cardiorespiratory function and the increase in body fat occurs partly because older individuals lead less active lives—not because of aging itself. If you maintain an active lifestyle, you can slow down the fitness decline seen in typical aging curves.

## What Risks Can Be Altered?

Many of the risks for heart disease (as well as for back problems) can be modified.

*Primary Risks.* Some characteristics and behaviors cause a higher risk for coronary heart disease (CHD) even in the absence of other risk factors. The independent, primary risk factors are

- smoking,
- high concentrations of serum low-density lipoprotein cholesterol (LDL-C),
- low concentrations of serum high-density lipoprotein cholesterol (HDL-C), and
- high blood pressure.

*Secondary Risks.* Some characteristics and behaviors cause increased risk of CHD only when other risk factors are present. In addition to the factors that cannot be altered (i.e., age, family history, gender, and race), there are other secondary risk factors:

- Physical inactivity
- Obesity
- High-fat diet
- Inability to cope with stress
- Coronary-prone personality
- High triglyceride levels

Though most reviewers consider inactivity, obesity, and a high-fat diet as secondary risk factors, there is increasing evidence that they are primary risk factors.

## How Does the Low Back Enter Into Fitness?

A healthy low back is an important component of fitness. Many fitness activities are impossible to pursue if back problems are present. Clinical evidence indicates that there are several risk factors associated with the development of low back problems:

- Lack of abdominal muscle endurance
- Lack of flexibility in the midtrunk and back of thighs
- Poor posture—lying, sitting, standing, moving
- Poor lifting habits
- Inability to cope with stress

## What Are Intelligent Goals for Me?

Research shows that you can enhance your health with regular physical activity, a well-rounded and nutritious diet, maintenance of recommended levels of body fat (through exercise and diet), learning to cope with stressors, and the ability to enjoy life without smoking, excess alcohol, or use of other drugs.

Fitness also includes unique aspects for each individual dependent on particular interests and aims in life. Maintaining certain body positions and postures for extended periods of time or varying the levels and types of physical activity may be a part of one's vocation. The things you enjoy doing during leisure time may also have different physical characteristics and requirements. Thus your plans for a healthier life should include not only the healthy behaviors essential for everyone but also specific activities designed to benefit your regular activities at work, at home, and during leisure.

## Can I Gain Control Over My Health Status?

The knowledge that you can modify your health status and risk of major health problems is both exciting and frustrating. It is exciting because you see how you can gain control of your health. But, it is frustrating in that you may find it difficult to change unhealthy lifestyles.

Starting a fitness program puts you at the cutting edge of health. We want to help you gain control of your life, beginning with an evaluation of risk factors and behaviors related to health. Chapter 2 deals with this type of health appraisal.

## Summary

Physical fitness is defined as those aspects of an ultimate quality of life that are related to positive physical health. Physical fitness is a necessary ingredient of total fitness, but total fitness includes much more than the physical aspects. You cannot achieve total fitness without a good physical health base. On the other hand, living with a high level of physical fitness but without the other aspects of fitness could prove to be a sterile existence. The relationship between physical fitness, health, and performance is depicted by describing the different goals of being free from disease, being able to do daily tasks efficiently, and competing in specific activities at desired skill levels. This chapter has dealt with risk factors that are associated with heart disease as well as the risk factors associated with low back problems that can and cannot be altered. Recognizing the characteristics and behaviors associated with health problems is the first step in gaining personal control over the factors contributing to good or poor health.

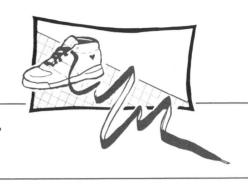

## Chapter
### 2

# *What Is My Health Status?*

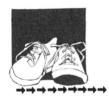

> **What Are My Known Health Problems?**
>
> **What Health-Related Characteristics/Signs/Symptoms Do I Have?**
>
> **What Healthy and Unhealthy Behaviors Do I Exhibit?**
>
> **How Can I Evaluate Test Scores Related to Health?**

The first step in starting a fitness program is to determine your current health status. Health status includes five major categories:

- Diagnosed medical problems
- Characteristics that increase the risk of health problems
- Signs or symptoms indicative of health problems
- Lifestyle behaviors related to positive or negative health
- Scores on physical fitness tests

You should now complete the Health Status Questionnaire (Table 2.1) to provide information about your health status (Figure 2.1).

The following sections will help you focus on different aspects of your health and fitness status.

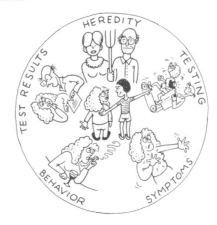

**Figure 2.1** Health status.

## Table 2.1
# Health Status Questionnaire

This key will assist you in using the information on this form. See text for further information.

EI   = Emergency Information. Be sure this is readily available to the fitness leader or your exercise partner.

MC   = Medical Clearance. Do not exercise without your physician's permission.

SEP  = Special Emergency Procedures. Do not exercise alone; make sure that your exercise partner knows what to do in case of an emergency.

PRF  = Primary Risk Factor for heart disease—ED needed.

SRF  = Secondary Risk Factor for heart disease—ED needed.

SLA  = Special or Limited Activities may be needed. You may need to include or exclude specific exercises; if unsure, check with your fitness leader or physician.

ED   = Educational Materials. You may want to get educational material or attend a workshop on this topic; check with your fitness leader or local health center for more information.

### Instructions

Complete *each* question accurately. All information provided is confidential if you choose to submit this form to your fitness instructor.

### Part 1. Information About the Individual

1. _____
   Social Sec. No.                                          Date _____

2. _____
   Legal name                                               Nickname _____

3. _____
   Mailing address                                          Home phone _____

                                                            Business phone _____

4. *EI* _____
   Personal physician                                       Phone _____

   Address _____

5. *EI* _____
   Person to contact in emergency                           Phone _____

6. *SRF* Gender (circle one):     Female     Male (*SRF*)

7. *SRF* Date of Birth: _____
                        Month                Day                Year

8. Number of hours worked per week:     Less than 20     20-40     41-60     Over 60

9. *SLA* More than 25% of time spent on job (circle all that apply)
   Sitting at desk     Lifting or carrying loads     Standing     Walking     Driving

### Part 2. Medical History

10. *SRF* Circle any who died of heart attack before age 50:
    Father          Mother          Brother          Sister          Grandparent

11. Date of
    Last medical physical exam: _____
                                Year

    Last physical fitness test: _____
                                Year

12. Circle operations you have had:

Back *SLA*       Heart *MC*       Kidney *SLA*       Other _____

Ears *SLA*       Hernia *SLA*       Lung *SLA*

Eyes *SLA*       Joint *SLA*       Neck *SLA*

13. Please circle any of the following for which you have been diagnosed or treated by a physician or health professional:

Alcoholism *SEP*                  Diabetes *SEP*                  Kidney problem *MC*

Anemia, sickle cell *SEP*         Emphysema *SEP*                 Mental illness *SEP*

Anemia, other *SEP*              Epilepsy *SEP*                  Neck strain *SLA*

Asthma SEP                       Eye problems *SLA*             Obesity *SRF*

Back strain *SLA*                Gout *SLA*                     Phlebitis *MC*

Bleeding trait *SEP*             Hearing loss *SLA*             Rheumatoid arthritis *SLA*

Bronchitis, chronic SEP          Heart problem *MC*             Stroke *MC*

Cancer *SEP*                     High blood pressure PRF        Thyroid problem SEP

Cirrhosis, liver *MC*            Hypoglycemia *SEP*             Ulcer *SEP*

Concussion *MC*                  Hyperlipidemia *PRF*           Other _____

Congenital defect *SEP*          Infectious mononucleosis *MC*

14. *ED* for all. Circle all medicine taken in last six months:

Blood thinner *MC*        Epilepsy medication *SEP*        Nitroglycerin *MC*

Diabetic pill SEP         Heart rhythm medication *MC*     Other _____

Digitalis *MC*            High blood pressure medication *MC*

Diuretic *MC*             Insulin *MC*

15. Any of these health symptoms that occurs frequently is the basis for medical attention. Circle the number indicating how often you have each of the following:

5 = Very often    2 = Infrequently
4 = Fairly often  1 = Practically never
3 = Sometimes

a. Cough up blood *MC*

   1    2    3    4    5

f. Chest pain *MC*

   1    2    3    4    5

b. Abdominal pain *MC*

   1    2    3    4    5

g. Swollen joints MC

   1    2    3    4    5

c. Low back pain *SLA*

   1    2    3    4    5

h. Feel faint *MC*

   1    2    3    4    5

d. Leg pain *MC*

   1    2    3    4    5

i. Dizziness *MC*

   1    2    3    4    5

e. Arm or shoulder pain *MC*

   1    2    3    4    5

j. Breathless with slight exertion *MC*

   1    2    3    4    5

(Cont.)

**Health Status Questionnaire (Continued)**

*Part 3. Health-Related Behavior*

16. *PRF* Do you now smoke?     Yes     No

17. If you are a smoker, indicate number smoked per day:

    Cigarettes:     40 or more          20-39          10-19          1-9

    Cigars or pipes only:     5 or more or any inhaled          Less than 5, none inhaled

18. *SRF* Do you exercise regularly?     Yes     No

19. How many days per week do you normally spend at least 20 minutes in moderate to strenuous exercise?

    0  1  2  3  4  5  6  7   days per week

20. Can you walk 4 miles briskly without fatigue?     Yes     No

21. Can you jog 3 miles continuously at a moderate pace without discomfort?     Yes     No

22. Weight now: _____ lbs.  One year ago: _____ lbs.  Age 21: _____ lbs.

*Part 4. Health-Related Attitudes*

23. *SRF* (Stress has been associated with coronary problems.) Circle the number that corresponds to how you feel:

    6 = Strongly agree
    5 = Moderately agree
    4 = Slightly agree
    3 = Slightly disagree
    2 = Moderately disagree
    1 = Strongly disagree

    I am an impatient, time-conscious, hard-driving individual

    1     2     3     4     5     6

24. List everything not already included on this questionnaire that might cause you problems in a fitness test or fitness program:

*Note.* Adapted from Howley and Franks (1986).

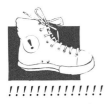

!!!!!!!!!!!!!!

## What Are My Known Health Problems?

Questions 12 to 14 should remind you of your known health problems that may affect your exercise program.

If you checked any of the items in Questions 12 to 14, you will need to work closely with the fitness director and your physician to ensure that you are involved in physical activities that are healthy for you. If you are on medication, changing your exercise habits requires close monitoring of medication levels and may involve some changes as you work with your physician and fitness leader.

## Which of My Characteristics Are Health-Related?

As we mentioned in chapter 1, you have a higher risk of cardiovascular disease if you had relatives (especially parents, Question 10) who died prior to age 50 from cardiovascular disease. You also have a higher risk if you are male and/or black. All of us have increased risk of major health problems as we grow older. Any of these characteristics should make you more determined to adopt healthy behaviors and change unhealthy practices.

## What Health-Related Signs/Symptoms Do I Have?

Question 15 on the Health Status Questionnaire includes some of the major signs and symptoms that could indicate a major health problem.

If you have any of these signs or symptoms, check with your physician to determine if they reflect a problem that needs medical attention. Do not begin a fitness program until you have discussed these signs and symptoms with a health care provider.

## What Are My Healthy and Unhealthy Behaviors?

Questions 16 to 23 and the ones you answered in chapter 1 are related to healthy (and unhealthy) behaviors. Your activities related to exercise, eating, smoking, use of alcohol and other drugs, and your ability to cope with stress are important elements in your health status.

## What Is the Relationship of Test Scores to Health?

If you are involved in a good fitness program, you will be taking a number of physical fitness tests as you go along. It is *not* important for you to perform better than *everyone else* on these tests, but it *is* important for you to be in the optimal range for percent body fat, have adequate levels of cardio-respiratory function, and develop sufficient abdominal strength/endurance and midtrunk flexibility to minimize the risks of low back problems. Ask your fitness leader to explain how your test results relate to health standards. If you are on a do-it-yourself fitness program, there are ways you can chart your progress. Can you walk, jog, or cycle at a moderate pace for longer periods without fatigue? Do everyday tasks such as climbing stairs, taking out the trash, or reaching for an object seem easier? If you had excess fat and have been doing fitness activities for several weeks, do you notice a difference in your waist size? Do you recover from physical exertion more easily? Do you have more energy late in the day? Are you sleeping better? Do you feel better after your workout than you did before the exercise? A good fitness program results in your answering *yes* to many of these questions.

## Summary

One of your first steps in starting a fitness program is to evaluate your current health status. This chapter provided you with information and a series of steps to begin that evaluation. It helped you identify your known medical problems. You should be aware of your personal characteristics that put you at risk for major health problems. The chapter referred to a number of signs, symptoms, and behaviors that are related to the healthy life. Finally, a few simple self-tests were included to assist you in your health status evaluation.

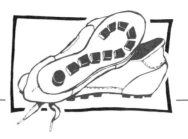

*Chapter*
**3**

# Should I Begin a Fitness Program?

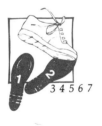

What Steps Should I Take to Get Started?

Does My Health Status Affect My Fitness Program?

What Kind of Fitness Program Should I Begin?

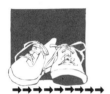

When most folks decide that they want to begin a fitness program, they think immediately of what activities they will do. Fitness activities, however, are only one part of a comprehensive fitness program; participation in fitness activities is preceded by other important steps. The different aspects of a fitness program are listed in Table 3.1.

**Table 3.1**
**Components of a Fitness Program**

Sequence of decisions for fitness

1. Deciding to do something
2. Determining health status
3. Seeking professional advice
4. Selecting a fitness program
5. Additional screening
6. Fitness testing
7. Fitness activities
8. Periodic testing
9. Modification of fitness activities

fitness program director. Since some variables may be influenced by your pretest activities and your reaction to the testing situation itself (some people are not used to being tested), borderline scores, especially at rest and during light activity, should be replicated before medical referral. For example, if you had a high resting heart rate or blood pressure, it may have been because you ate, smoked, took medicine, or participated in physical exercise just prior to the test. Were you anxious about taking the test itself? Were there unusual conditions during the test (lots of people, noise, etc.)? The exercise leader may have you rest for a few minutes, reassure you about the purpose and safety of the test, and test you again. Or you may be rescheduled for another day. If the questionable test result is repeated, then you can be referred to a health care specialist.

Other factors may indicate that a person with the characteristics we have listed as warranting a "supervised" program should actually be medically referred; for example, having multiple risk factors, each close to the referral value. Or the medical consultant may recommend that someone in our "refer" category enter a supervised program, based on a recent medical examination or conversation with the personal physician. Programs with excellent and accessible medical and emergency personnel may use higher values for referral than do programs isolated from medical and emergency facilities.

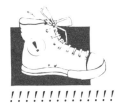

!!!!!!!!!!!!!!

### Should I Be in a Supervised Program?

Table 3.3 lists conditions that, if severe, may be the basis for medical referral. If you have mild or moderate levels, however, you can participate in a carefully supervised fitness program. It is important that the exercise leader be informed of these or other conditions that may be related to your ability to exercise.

**Table 3.3**
**Basis for a Supervised Program:**
**Recently Diagnosed or Treated Medical Conditions**

| | |
|---|---|
| Alcoholism | Diabetes |
| Allergy | Emphysema |
| Anemia | Epilepsy |
| Asthma | Hypoglycemia |
| Bleeding trait | Mental illness |
| Bronchitis | Peptic ulcer |
| Cancer | Pregnancy |
| Colitis | Thyroid problem |

### What May Need Special Attention?

Table 3.4 lists numerous problems that call for special or limited activities.

### Can I Participate in All Fitness Activities?

If you have none of the health problems, conditions, or behaviors we've listed that require medical referral or supervised programs; have no questionable responses to fitness tests; and have no other reason to question your ability to continue physical activities, then you can participate in any of the fitness

**Table 3.4**
**Basis for Special Attention**

| Large amounts of time spent | Operations | Other problems |
| --- | --- | --- |
| Driving | Back | Arthritis |
| Lifting | Eyes | Eye problems |
| Sitting | Joint(s) | Gout |
| Standing | Lungs | Hearing loss |
| | Neck | Hernia |
| | | Low back pain |

activities in this book, using the recommended levels of work, with minimal risk. Your major goals will be to improve or maintain your fitness level through activities that provide an appropriate fitness stimulus and are enjoyable to you. You may want to try some new activities to add variety to your work-outs.

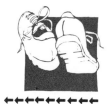

## Summary

Chapter 2 helped you evaluate your current health status. This chapter helped you use that information to decide on a safe and appropriate fitness program. The health status form and suggested fitness test items identify characteristics that should cause you to check with your personal physician before starting an exercise program. If you have any doubt about your health status, that step is recommended. This chapter also helped you distinguish among those conditions and risk factors that would be the basis for beginning your fitness activities in a program that is supervised by a qualified fitness instructor. Finally, the chapter provided you with the information to determine if you can begin your own exercise program with minimal health risks.

# *WHAT SHOULD I DO TO BE FIT?*

**How Much Should I Weigh?**

**What Should My Cardiorespiratory Fitness Level Be?**

**How Can I Prevent Low Back Problems?**

**How Can I Cope With Stressors?**

Part 1 helped you evaluate your current health status. This section of the book deals with recommendations concerning the various elements of physical fitness.

Chapter 4 assists you in evaluating your body fat and determining your optimal range of body weight. Chapter 5 helps you select a healthy diet. Chapter 6 helps you understand the tests of aerobic (cardiorespiratory) fitness. Chapters 7 and 8 deal with total body muscular strength/endurance and flexibility. Chapter 9 provides information concerning low back pain, which is a real or potential problem for all of us. Chapter 10 outlines ways to maximize the positive and minimize the negative aspects of stress in our lives.

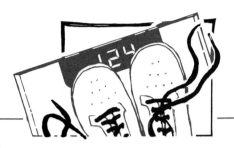

## Chapter
### 4

# *How Much Should I Weigh?*

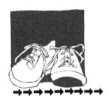

→+→+→+→+→+

---

**How Do I Determine My Optimal Weight?**
**How Do I Change the Amount of Fat I Have?**
**How Can Exercise Help With Weight Control?**

---

Many Americans have a full-time preoccupation with losing weight. Part of the reason for this is due to social pressure to have a certain "look," but part is related to the health consequences of carrying too much fat. People who are too fat are more likely to have high blood pressure, heart disease, and diabetes. The purpose of this chapter is to help you separate fact from fiction with regard to body composition and weight control.

## How Do I Analyze My Weight?

The human body is composed of a wide variety of tissues and organs such as muscle, bone, heart, liver, brain, and fat. To simplify our discussion of body composition, we will divide the body into lean mass and fat mass and express each as a percent of total body weight. For example, a man who is 20% fat and weighs 200 pounds is carrying 40 pounds of fat (20% of 200 pounds). Lean mass includes all tissues and organs other than fat. Fat mass includes *essential fat* (fat that is necessary for survival), and the "extra" that we carry along. Fat is found in all cells, surrounds most nerves, and is associated with specific tissues. Essential fat totals about 3% of body weight for men and 12% of body weight for women. The higher value for women allows for the fat that is usually deposited in the breasts and hips at puberty and is related to the hormone estrogen. It is important that you understand the nature of essential fat because it sets the lower limit of body fatness for men and women.

What, then, is a reasonable amount of fat? Body fatness values associated with good health are *neither too low nor too high*. In the past most fitness books were concerned solely with too much fat; that is no longer true. Our country has experienced an increase in the number of feeding-disorder problems associated with people (primarily teenage girls and young women) who have a drive to be as thin as possible. *Anorexia nervosa* is an eating disorder in which people have a distorted view of their body fatness; they see themselves as fat even if they are emaciated. *Bulimia* describes a ritual of overeating followed by vomiting to help keep body weight low. Concern about feeding disorders has led to the identification of both low and high body fatness values that are consistent with good health.

Further, you should recognize that recommended body fatness values will be different for the athlete interested in world-class performance than for the average person participating in a health-related fitness program. Figure 4.1 lists body fatness values that bracket the healthy range. Your goal should be to achieve the optimal range. Keep in mind the fact that body fatness normally fluctuates some amount during the year, as physical activity and food consumption patterns vary with the season and holidays.

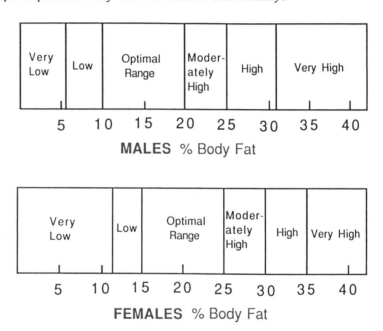

**Figure 4.1**  Body fatness values. *Note*. Adapted from Lohman (1987).

## How Is Body Fatness Determined?

Body fatness can be evaluated by a wide variety of techniques; this section will discuss only the most common. We will start by excluding some, then recommend others.

The "mirror test," in which you stand naked in front of a full-length mirror, requires strict objectivity to discern what is too little and what is too much as far as fat is concerned. Although it is not a bad idea to take a look at ourselves in this way every once in a while, we can sometimes fool ourselves into thinking we are just right when we are in fact fat or think we are too fat when we are actually very thin, as in the case of anorexia nervosa.

One of the most common, but limited, ways to analyze body composition is the height/weight table. The Metropolitan Life Insurance Company has provided such tables to show "ideal" weights that are related to a low death rate in adults. Table 4.1 shows their norms for men and women of different

**Table 4.1**
**Desirable Weights for Men and Women, 25 Years of Age and Over**

| Height[a] | | Small frame | Medium frame | Large frame |
|---|---|---|---|---|
| Feet | Inches | | | |
| | | Men | | |
| 5 | 2 | 112-120 | 118-129 | 126-141 |
| 5 | 3 | 115-123 | 121-133 | 129-144 |
| 5 | 4 | 118-126 | 124-136 | 132-148 |
| 5 | 5 | 121-129 | 127-139 | 135-152 |
| 5 | 6 | 124-133 | 130-143 | 138-156 |
| 5 | 7 | 128-137 | 134-147 | 142-161 |
| 5 | 8 | 132-141 | 138-152 | 147-166 |
| 5 | 9 | 136-145 | 142-156 | 151-170 |
| 5 | 10 | 140-150 | 146-160 | 155-174 |
| 5 | 11 | 144-154 | 150-165 | 159-179 |
| 6 | 0 | 148-158 | 154-170 | 164-184 |
| 6 | 1 | 152-162 | 158-175 | 168-189 |
| 6 | 2 | 156-167 | 162-180 | 173-194 |
| 6 | 3 | 160-171 | 167-185 | 178-199 |
| 6 | 4 | 164-175 | 172-190 | 182-204 |
| | | Women | | |
| 4 | 10 | 92- 98 | 96-107 | 104-119 |
| 4 | 11 | 94-101 | 98-110 | 106-122 |
| 5 | 0 | 96-104 | 101-113 | 109-125 |
| 5 | 1 | 99-107 | 104-116 | 112-128 |
| 5 | 2 | 102-110 | 107-119 | 115-131 |
| 5 | 3 | 105-113 | 110-122 | 118-134 |
| 5 | 4 | 108-116 | 113-126 | 121-138 |
| 5 | 5 | 111-119 | 116-130 | 125-142 |
| 5 | 6 | 114-123 | 120-135 | 129-146 |
| 5 | 7 | 118-127 | 124-139 | 133-150 |
| 5 | 8 | 122-131 | 128-143 | 137-154 |
| 5 | 9 | 126-135 | 132-147 | 141-158 |
| 5 | 10 | 130-140 | 136-151 | 145-163 |
| 5 | 11 | 134-144 | 140-155 | 149-168 |
| 6 | 0 | 138-148 | 144-159 | 153-173 |

*Note.* From "New Weight Standards for Men and Women" by the Metropolitan Life Insurance Company of New York, 1959 *Statistical Bulletin,* **40**, pp. 1-4. Courtesy *Statistical Bulletin*; Metropolitan Life Insurance Co.

[a]For men, height includes shoes with 1-inch heels; for women, 2-inch heels.

heights and frame sizes. There is a range of weights for any frame size, but as Figure 4.2 shows, as a person becomes fatter it is *easy* to move up a frame size to accommodate that increased body weight! If you are 10% above the ideal weight (midpoint of the weight range at any height), you are classified as overweight; if 20% above ideal, you are classified as obese. There are at least two concerns that can be raised about height/weight tables: How do you determine your frame size, and how does simple body weight indicate how fat you are? The latter question is the most important limitation in the use of these tables. Many highly trained football players who are large and lean would be classified as obese by these tables, because the simple measure of

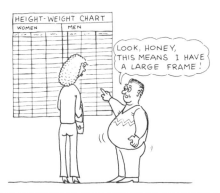

**Figure 4.2** One way to interpret the height/weight chart.

body weight does not distinguish between lean tissue and fat tissue. For this reason, these tables are not recommended for use in the evaluation of body composition.

The two recommended ways to analyze body composition are shown in Figure 4.3. *Underwater weighing*, also known as hydrostatic weighing, measures body density, the tendency of a person to sink when placed in water. With this technique your weight is measured on land with a calibrated scale and again when you are completely submerged underwater. The idea is that, because fat tends to float, a lean person will weigh more underwater than a fat person. For example, if we measured underwater weights on two people, each weighing 200 pounds, the person with the lower body density would weigh less. On the basis of the land and underwater weights the density and relative fatness of the body are calculated. This technique is accurate but time-consuming and doing it correctly requires special equipment and personnel. This makes it an expensive way to determine body fatness, and it is not commonly used.

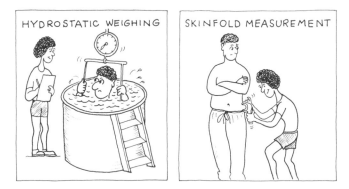

**Figure 4.3** Methods of determining body fatness.

The most common method of evaluating body composition is by measuring the thickness of several skinfolds. This technique relies on the observation that a large amount of the total body fat is located just under the skin, and by obtaining an estimate of that fat, overall body fatness can be determined.

If you are in a good fitness program, you have probably had your percent fat estimated by underwater weighing or skinfold measurements. If you are not in a fitness program and want to determine your percent fat and how much you should lose or gain, check with a fitness program in your area. You will know, of course, that your fat levels are changing when you notice that your clothes fit you differently.

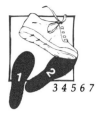

# How Can I Estimate My Percent Fat?

We encourage you to have your percent fat determined by underwater weighing or by skinfold site measurements by fitness professionals. However, you can make a rough estimate of percent fat.

*Women* can estimate their percent fat in the following way:

1. Determine standing height (without shoes) in inches.
2. Measure hip girth at the widest point in inches.
3. Go to Figure 4.4 and draw a straight line from hip girth measurement (on the left) to standing height (on the right).
4. Find the point where the line crosses the middle scale—this is the estimated percent fat.

For example, a woman with a hip girth of 36 inches who is 60 inches (5 feet) tall has an estimated percent fat of 26% (determined by drawing a line from 36 on the left to 60 on the right and finding that it crosses the percent fat scale at 26).

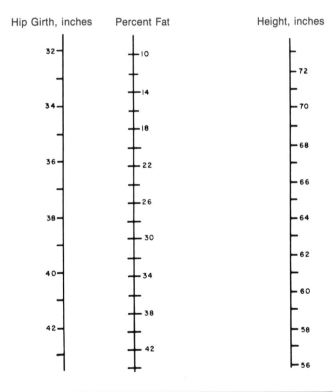

**Figure 4.4** Estimation of relative fat in women from height and hip circumference. *Note.* Adapted from Wilmore (1986).

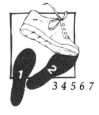

*Men* can estimate their percent fat in the following way:

1. Determine weight in pounds.
2. Measure waist girth at the widest point in inches.
3. Go to Figure 4.5 and draw a straight line from body weight (on the left) to waist girth (on the right).
4. Find the point where the line crosses the middle scale—that is the estimated percent fat. For example, a man who weighs 200 pounds with a waist girth of 40 inches has an estimated percent fat of 26%.

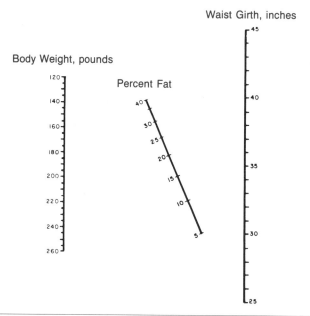

Figure 4.5 Estimation of relative fat in men from body weight and abdominal or waist circumference. *Note.* Adapted from Wilmore (1986).

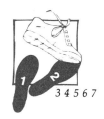

## How Can I Calculate Target Weight Range?

You can determine your desired weight using the estimated percent fat (either from testing at a fitness center or by the above method). This is a better way of deciding your optimal weight than simply using a height/weight chart, because this method is based on how much fat you should have.

1. Weigh yourself to get your current body weight: _____ pounds

2. Record the percent body fat: _____ %

3. Multiply your percent body fat, converted to a decimal value, by your body weight to yield fat weight:

   Body fat 0._____ times body weight pounds = _____ pounds fat weight

4. Subtract this fat weight from your total body weight to yield lean body weight:

   Body weight _____ pounds minus fat weight _____ pounds

   = _____ pounds lean weight

5. Divide lean weight by 0.80 to 0.90 (allowing for 10 to 20% ideal body fatness for men), or by .75 to .85 (15 to 25% body fat for women). (Note: Remember that .80 lean weight corresponds with .20 fat weight; .90 lean weight, .10 fat weight; and so forth.) This is the target weight range.

For example:

1. If a man is 24% fat and weighs 189 pounds, his fat weight is 45.4 pounds (.24 times 189 pounds = 45.4 pounds).
2. Subtracting 45.4 pounds from 189 pounds leaves 143.6 pounds for lean body weight.
3. His ideal body fatness range is 10 to 20%, so divide 143.6 pounds by .80 and by .90 to yield 160 to 180 pounds as his target weight range.

4. Try to achieve the upper part of the range at a rate of 1 pound every 2 weeks (in this example, a loss of 9 pounds from 189 to 180 within 18 weeks).

## How Do I Change My Fat Level?

The previous sections have described the difference between body weight and body fat and showed you how to estimate body fatness by very simple procedures. This section deals with the issues related to changing body weight and body composition.

### What About Caloric Balance and Weight Control?

When we discuss weight control and body composition, we are dealing with the issues of gaining and losing fat and lean tissue. There is no question that body weight can be lost through excessive sweating or with the use of diuretic drugs that cause the kidneys to produce lots of urine. However, water weight is easily replaced and has no effect on the fat weight that is linked to diabetes and heart disease. Therefore, in our discussion of this topic we will refer only to methods that alter the fat mass and the lean mass of the body; in this way body composition can be altered to improve health status.

The central concept related to weight control is found in the *energy balance equation*:

---

**If caloric intake *is equal to* caloric expenditure, then energy balance exists → no change in weight**

**If caloric intake *is greater than* caloric expenditure, then positive energy balance exists → weight gain**

**If caloric intake *is less than* caloric expenditure, then negative energy balance exists → weight loss**

---

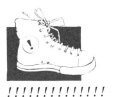

*!!!!!!!!!!!!!!*

Caloric intake refers to the number of kilocalories (kcal) of food that are consumed, and caloric expenditure refers to the total number of kcal that are expended at rest, during work, and as a result of exercise. In everyday usage, a kilocalorie is called simply a calorie. (Chapter 13 provides estimates of daily caloric expenditures for different activity levels.) If you wish to maintain your body weight you must balance intake and expenditure, and *if you wish to lose weight you must create a negative energy balance by expending more calories than you consume.*

This negative energy balance can be accomplished by keeping your energy expenditure the same and reducing your caloric intake. In this case, the focus of attention is on trying to eat a nutritionally sound diet while consuming fewer calories (kcal). You can also achieve a weight loss by keeping your diet the same but increasing your energy expenditure. In either case, you must lose *3,500 kcal* from your body's energy store to lose 1 pound of fat. If you were to create a negative energy balance of 500 kcal per day you would lose about 1 pound of fat per week. The recommended rate of weight loss is a *maximum* of 1 to 2 pounds per week, so the total negative energy balance should be no more than about 1,000 kcal per day. We recommend more modest changes in diet and exercise to achieve a loss of 1 pound every two weeks.

### How Does Exercise Affect Appetite?

At first thought, it seems that if you exercise more you will eat more, lessening exercise's effect on weight. People who begin moderate exercise programs, however, show little or no changes in appetite. Most people can do fitness workouts of 30 to 60 minutes several days per week without increasing their caloric intakes. Some individuals find that they are not as hungry and eat less when they are active on a regular basis.

### What About Diet, Exercise, and Cholesterol?

Proper exercise and diet affect more than weight loss. It has been shown that a low-fat diet that contains only 30% fat (like the one discussed in the next chapter) is associated with low levels of serum cholesterol, one of the major risk factors of heart disease. In addition, exercise appears to have a separate effect of raising the level of "good" high-density lipoprotein (HDL) cholesterol. The result of lowering total cholesterol and raising HDL cholesterol is to reduce the risk of heart disease.

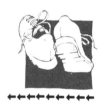

## Summary

You should strive for a healthy level of body fat, which is between 10 and 20% for men and between 15 and 25% for women. Your body fatness and your target weight range can be estimated from skinfold or girth measurements. Excess body fat can best be reduced by modest changes in exercise and dietary patterns, resulting in a loss of one pound of fat (negative caloric balance of 3,500 kcal) every 2 weeks.

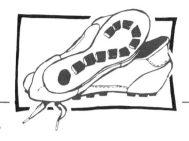

*Chapter*
**5**

# What Is a Healthy Food Plan?

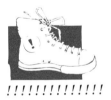

➔➔➔➔➔➔➔➔

---

**What Should I Eat?**

**What Should I Avoid Eating?**

---

There is no question that caloric intake is one of the factors in our weight loss equation. However, a food plan, commonly called a diet, involves more than just calories. The types of food we eat have a major bearing on overall health and well-being. This section will present some basic information relative to diet and the nutritional goals we should try to achieve.

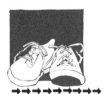

!!!!!!!!!!!!!!

## What Should I Eat?

We now have clear evidence that the typical American diet has adversely affected our health. There are clear links between overconsumption of saturated fats and cholesterol and the rate of heart disease in this country. In addition, lack of dietary fiber has been tied to a variety of intestinal health problems. Because of this information, the United States Senate Select Commission on Nutrition and Human Needs held hearings in 1977 to determine dietary goals that would point the way toward improved health status for U.S. citizens. The outcome of these deliberations is shown in Figure 5.1. The left side of the figure shows current dietary patterns, and the right side lists the goals.

In general, the recommendations call for

- increasing carbohydrate intake (46 to 58% of total diet) while simultaneously decreasing intake of simple sugars,
- decreasing total (42 to 30%) and saturated (16 to 10%) fat intake, limiting cholesterol to 300 milligrams per day, and
- reducing salt consumption by about 50 to 85% to only 3 grams per day.

You will find a more detailed explanation of these recommendations in the next section of this chapter.

food intake is protein, which is sufficient to meet this standard. The Senate committee's dietary goals recommend no change in this quantity but suggest that to keep the intake of fat at a lower level, Americans should eat more fish, poultry, and low-fat dairy products rather than red meat and regular milk products.

*Vitamins* are a class of special nutrients that are required in very small amounts but are vitally necessary for normal function. They are classified as *fat soluble* or *water soluble* based on their ability to dissolve in lipids or in water. Fat-soluble vitamins include A, D, E, and K. Because of their solubility, they can be stored in the body and are not needed every day since you can "catch up" on other days.

A potential problem with fat-soluble vitamins is that if you take in too much of them over a long period of time, you can actually develop hypervitaminosis, a toxicity condition that can lead to nervous disorders, gastrointestinal problems, and damage to your liver and kidneys. Water-soluble vitamins, which include the B vitamins, C, folic acid, pantothenic acid, and biotin, are much less likely to induce hypervitaminosis, since any excess is excreted in the urine. However, high levels of water-soluble vitamins can be toxic and should also be avoided. Due to the high turnover of water-soluble vitamins, you need to replace your supplies of them on a daily basis. A summary of these vitamins, their function, and their food sources are presented in Table 5.1. The last two columns of the table list the adult requirements for each vitamin. These values are taken from the Tables of Recommended Dietary Allowances (RDA) and Estimated Safe and Adequate Daily Dietary Intakes found in Appendixes A and B. These values are consistent with the requirements of healthy people. Requirements are different for men, children, women, and pregnant or lactating women. Though these are the values with which you can evaluate the adequacy of your diet, do not expect to meet each requirement on a daily basis. Evaluate your diet over a period of several days to see if, on the average, your intake is adequate.

Should you take a vitamin supplement? You can meet the daily requirements for all vitamins by eating a varied diet containing the four food groups (discussion follows), and if you are doing so, you do not need a vitamin supplement. If you want to make sure you're getting all the vitamins, taking a single multivitamin every other day will generally not cause problems. On the other hand, it is better to focus your attention on eating a balanced diet to meet these needs in the long run than depending on a supplement. Remember, by eating a balanced diet, you also fulfill protein and mineral requirements.

*Minerals* are chemical elements that, like vitamins, are needed in small amounts for normal health. Minerals are divided into two classes: *major minerals* and *trace minerals*. Major minerals include calcium for bones, potassium and sodium for nerve and muscle function, and magnesium that is needed for many of the body's enzymes to function. Trace minerals include iron for hemoglobin that is needed to transport oxygen in the blood; iodine for the hormone thyroxine that is needed to keep our metabolic rates at the right level; and zinc, selenium, copper, and others that are needed for certain enzymes to function properly. You can achieve the daily requirements for most of these minerals by eating a varied and balanced diet. However, there is some concern that women do not take in sufficient amounts of iron and calcium; women may opt for supplementation of these minerals. Table 5.2 presents a summary of the major and trace minerals, food sources, and adult requirements.

**Table 5.1**
**Vitamins and Their Functions**

| Vitamin | Function | Sources | Daily adult requirement[a] | |
|---|---|---|---|---|
| | | | Men | Women |
| Thiamin (B-1) | Functions as part of a coenzyme to aid utilization of energy | Whole grains, nuts, lean pork | 1.4 mg[b] | 1.0 mg |
| Riboflavin (B-2) | Involved in energy metabolism as part of a coenzyme | Milk, yogurt, cheese | 1.6 mg | 1.2 mg |
| Niacin | Facilitates energy production in cells | Lean meat, fish, poultry, grains | 18.0 mg | 13.0 mg |
| Vitamin B-6 | Absorbs and metabolizes protein; aids in red blood cell formation | Lean meat, vegetables, whole grains | 2.2 mg | 2.0 mg |
| Pantothenic acid | Aids in metabolism of carbohydrate, fat, and protein | Whole-grain cereals, bread, dark green vegetables | 4 - 7 mg | 4 - 7 mg |
| Folic acid | Functions as coenzyme in synthesis of nucleic acids and protein | Green vegetables, beans, whole-wheat products | 400 µg | 400 µg |
| Vitamin B-12 | Involved in synthesis of nucleic acids, red blood cell formation | Only in animal foods, not plant foods | 3 µg | 3 µg |
| Biotin | Coenzyme in synthesis of fatty acids and glycogen formation | Egg yolk, dark green vegetables | 1 - 200 µg | 1 - 200 µg |
| C | Intracellular maintenance of bone, capillaries, and teeth | Citrus fruits, green peppers, tomatoes | 60 mg | 60 mg |
| A | Functions in visual processes; formation and maintenance of skin and mucous membranes | Carrots, sweet potatoes, margarine, butter, liver | 5,000 IU | 5,000 IU |
| D | Aids in growth and formation of bones and teeth; promotes calcium absorption | Eggs, tuna, liver, fortified milk | 5 mg | 5 mg |
| E | Protects polyunsaturated fats; prevents cell membrane damage | Vegetable oils, whole-grain cereal and bread, green leafy vegetables | 10 mg | 8 mg |
| K | Important in blood clotting | Green leafy vegetables, peas, potatoes | 70 - 140 µg | 70 - 140 µg |

*Note.* Adapted from Howley and Franks (1986).

[a]Values are for adults 23 to 50 years of age. The requirements vary for children and pregnant or lactating women. See Appendixes A and B.

[b]mg = milligram, µg = microgram, IU = international unit.

**Table 5.2
Minerals and Their Functions**

| Mineral | Function | Sources | Daily adult requirement[a] | |
| --- | --- | --- | --- | --- |
| | | | Men | Women |
| *Major minerals* | | | | |
| Calcium | Bones, teeth, blood clotting, nerve and muscle function | Milk, sardines, dark green vegetables, nuts | 800 mg | 800-1500 mg[b] |
| Chloride | Nerve and muscle function, water balance (with sodium) | Table salt | 1.7-5.1 g | 1.7-5.1 g |
| Magnesium | Bone growth; nerve, muscle, and enzyme function | Nuts, seafood, whole grains, leafy green vegetables | 350 mg | 300 mg |
| Phosphorus | Bone, teeth, energy transfer | Meats, poultry, seafood, eggs, milk, beans | 800 mg | 800 mg |
| Potassium | Nerve and muscle function | Fresh vegetables, bananas, citrus fruits, milk, meats, fish | 1875-5625 mg | 1875-5625 mg |
| Sodium | Nerve and muscle function, water balance | Table salt | 1.1-3.3 g | 1.1-3.3 g |
| *Trace minerals* | | | | |
| Chromium | Glucose metabolism | Meats, liver, whole grains, dried beans | .05-.2 mg | .05-.2 mg |
| Copper | Enzyme function, energy production | Meats, seafood, nuts, grains | 2-3 mg | 2-3 mg |
| Fluoride | Bone and teeth growth | Drinking water, fish, milk | 1.5-4 mg | 1.5-4 mg |
| Iodine | Thyroid hormone formation | Iodized salt, seafood | 150 mg | 150 mg |
| Iron | $O_2$ transport in red blood cells; enzyme function | Red meat, liver, eggs, beans, leafy vegetables, shell fish | 10 mg | 18 mg |
| Manganese | Enzyme function | Whole grains, nuts, fruits, vegetables | 2.5-5 mg | 2.5-5 mg |
| Molybdenum | Energy metabolism in cells | Whole grains, organ meats, peas, beans | .15-.5 mg | .15-.5 mg |
| Selenium | Works with vitamin E | Meat, fish, whole grains, eggs | .05-.2 mg | .05-.2 mg |
| Zinc | Part of enzymes, growth | Meat, shellfish, yeast, whole grains | 15 mg | 15 mg |

*Note.* Adapted from Christian and Greger (1985) and Williams (1988).

[a]Values are for adults 23 to 50 years of age. Requirements vary for children and pregnant or lactating women. See Appendixes A and B.

[b]For postmenopausal women, increase to 1200 to 1500 milligrams per day.

## How Do I Meet Dietary Requirements?

A variety of food plans can be followed to meet daily requirements for the various classes of nutrients. One of the most common is the Basic Four Food Group plan. This plan has been around a long time. Most school children are familiar with it as it is presented in health classes in the elementary grades. The basic four food groups include meat and meat substitutes, milk and milk products, fruits and vegetables, and grains. The focus of attention in this plan is on *nutrient density*. This means that the foods chosen from each group are high in selected nutrients—for example, protein and vitamins. Table 5.3 presents these food groups, sample foods and serving sizes, the number of adult servings required per day, and the major nutrients found in each food group. However, following this classic plan can still leave you short of some vitamins and minerals. Suggested modifications include eating 3 ounce portions of meat, not 2 to 3 ounces; adding two servings of legumes or nuts; making the grains "whole" grains; and adding one serving of fat or oil to provide vitamin E. Since this modification will increase caloric intake, emphasize using lean red meats, poultry, and fish for your meat group; trimming excess fat off meat; broiling rather than frying; and using low-fat dairy products. If these adjustments still cause you to take in more calories than you are expending, consider increasing your physical activity to cover the difference rather than cut back on food intake. In that way it will be easier for you to meet all nutrient requirements. The Basic Four Food Group plan emphasizes variety in pursuit of the balanced diet. By eating a variety of foods within each group you are more likely to meet the requirements over time. In addition, the emphasis on lean meats, fish, poultry, whole grains, low-fat dairy products, and lots of fruits and vegetables allows you to achieve the United

**Table 5.3**
**The Basic Four Food Group Plan**

| Food group | Sample foods and serving size | Number of daily servings for adults | Major nutrients |
|---|---|---|---|
| Meat and meat substitutes | 2-3 oz lean meat, fish, or poultry<br>2 eggs<br>1 cup cooked legumes<br>4 tablespoons peanut butter | 2 | Protein, iron, niacin, and riboflavin |
| Milk and milk products | 1 cup (8 fluid oz) milk or yogurt<br>2 cups cottage cheese<br>1.5 cups ice cream<br>1-2 oz cheese | 2 | Protein, calcium, riboflavin, zinc, vitamin D |
| Fruits and vegetables | ½ cup fruit; select from citrus fruits (vitamin C)<br>Dark green or yellow vegetables (vitamin A) | 4 | Vitamins A and C; carbohydrate |
| Grains (breads and cereal products) | 1 slice bread<br>1 oz ready-to-eat cereal<br>½-¾ cup cooked cereal, grits, macaroni, rice, noodles, or spaghetti | 4 | Carbohydrates; additional amounts of iron, thiamin, and niacin |

*Note.* Adapted from Hamilton and Whitney (1982).

- How long has your weight been what it is now? _____
- When you eat at home, who does the cooking? _____
- How often do you eat out? _____
  For what meals? _____

This fill-in-the-blank review gives you an idea of how your dietary habits compare to the recommendations mentioned earlier that aim at reducing fat intake and increasing consumption of complex carbohydrates. Further, by focusing attention on how you cook food, your likes and dislikes, your favorite snacks, and the circumstances surrounding when and where you eat, you can begin to control your caloric intake.

For example, if you always find yourself eating snacks in your easy chair watching television, there may be an association between the eating of the snack and the comfort of that TV room. It is clear that to change any habits, including dietary ones, you may first have to change the circumstances associated with the habit. If you restrict all your eating to the kitchen, you may find your eating habits easier to change. Additional details on how to change habits are presented in chapter 14.

## What Should I Avoid?

We have tried to present some basic, sound information relating diet to health and weight control. There is no question about the interest in this topic—just look at all the dietary books and programs for sale in every community. Unfortunately, but not surprisingly, some books and programs provide incorrect and potentially dangerous information regarding diet, exercise, and weight loss. The purpose of this section is to discuss these fads and gimmicks that are sold under the pretense that they will help a person achieve a weight loss goal.

The vast majority of people who lose weight regain it within a year because they have not dealt with the factors involved in the energy balance equation: energy expenditure and caloric intake. In addition, they have not paid attention to changing their lifestyle behaviors that are related to patterns of eating and exercise. It is generally recommended that you create a caloric imbalance of about 500 to 1,000 kcal per day through modifications in diet and exercise. This adjustment will cause the loss of about 1 or 2 pounds per week and allow you to gain control over exercise and eating behaviors. We cannot overemphasize the need to make *small and systematic changes* in your diet and activity levels to cause the weight loss and to maintain your new weight when you reach your goal. In the process you will learn how to plan meals better to meet the dietary goals and RDA standards. We have provided a checklist (Table 5.6) to help you make decisions about weight loss diets; the next time you are considering a diet, use the checklist to help you.

There is no lack of fad diets and commercial enterprises that promise an incredible weight loss in a short period of time. As we mentioned earlier, there is money to be made, and you need to be wary of exaggerated claims. The saying "If it's too good to be true, it probably is" is a good way to approach weight loss diets and gimmicks. We would like to comment on a few of the more common gimmicks used to "lose" weight.

- **Diuretics** These drugs cause sodium, potassium, and water loss from the body. The weight change that occurs as a result is therefore unrelated to body fatness.
- **Laxatives** These medications are usually used to loosen fecal matter in the large intestine and promote bowel movements. People who use laxa-

**Table 5.6**
**Weight Loss Diet Evaluation Checklist**

The following checklist can be used to evaluate weight loss diets. A *No* answer to any of the questions indicates an inadequate weight reduction plan. Does your diet

|  | Yes | No |
|---|---|---|
| 1. Aim for a weight loss of 1 to 2 pounds per week? | ☐ | ☐ |
| 2. Provide at least 1,200 kcal per day? | ☐ | ☐ |
| 3. Recommend a regular endurance exercise program? | ☐ | ☐ |
| 4. Provide a balance of foods from all four food groups? | ☐ | ☐ |
| 5. Provide for variety to prevent boredom? | ☐ | ☐ |
| 6. Establish eating and exercise habits that can be maintained the rest of your life? | ☐ | ☐ |
| 7. Conform to your personal lifestyle? | ☐ | ☐ |
| 8. Work without pills, drugs, or other gadgets? | ☐ | ☐ |

*Note.* From Howley and Franks (1986).

tives for weight loss are under the assumption that if laxatives speed things along the intestinal tract, some food will not be absorbed into the body. This is not true. Laxatives have little effect on absorption but instead cause the loss of important minerals and water from the body.

- **"Sauna" suits**   These suits are made of materials impermeable to sweat, which must be evaporated from the surface of the skin to cool the body during exercise. Because evaporation does not occur when these suits are worn, the body sweats more in an attempt to cool itself. This results in a loss of water weight that will (and must) be replaced as soon as possible. These suits do not "burn" calories away. Sitting in a "sauna" room has the same effect on water weight.

- **Elastic belts**   These belts are worn around the waist and allegedly "melt" fat away, causing changes in your waist size. As it turns out, your waist size does decrease because the tissues are compressed; within a few hours, however, the tissues return to their normal size and the effect disappears.

- **Vibrators or massagers**   These devices promise to break up fat in localized areas, cause "spot reduction," and speed weight loss. "Spot reduction" is a dream that can't come true because weight is lost from the body in a pattern opposite to the way it went on. If the fat went to your hips first and your face last, it will come from your face first and your hips last when you lose body fat. These machines may be enjoyable to use, but they do not increase energy expenditure, which is the necessary ingredient in weight loss.

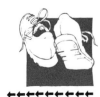

## Summary

The recommended food plan includes a balanced diet with 58% of calories coming from carbohydrates, no more than 30% from fat (less than 10% from saturated fat), and 12% from proteins. This calls for an increase in complex carbohydrates and a reduction in fat in the typical American diet. Specific recommendations for the changes in carbohydrates include *decreasing* consumption of soft drinks, cakes, cookies, and other high-sugar foods; and *increasing* intake of whole-grain breads, cereals, fruits, vegetables, and beans. Recommended ways of reducing fat include using low-fat milk, less and leaner meat, and using fish, poultry, and dry beans and peas as sources for proteins. Also, limit eggs and organ meats, as well as fats and oils, especially those high in saturated fats (e.g., butter; lard; palm and coconut oils). This chapter provided information about the basic four food groups and has outlined a system where similar foods can be substituted for each other to help you establish a healthy diet.

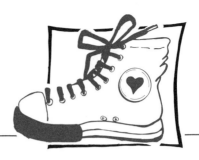

## Chapter 6

# What About Aerobic Fitness?

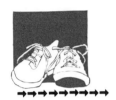

---

**What Tests Can I Use to Measure Aerobic Fitness?**

**How Can I Evaluate My Aerobic Fitness?**

---

Aerobic fitness is a good measure of your heart's ability to pump oxygen-rich blood to the muscles. This is also called cardiovascular or cardiorespiratory fitness (CRF). Although there are technical differences in terms using cardio (heart), vascular (blood vessels), respiratory (lungs), and aerobic (working with oxygen), they all reflect various aspects of this component of fitness. We will use these terms in a general way to represent this fitness area. The person with a healthy, large heart can pump great volumes of blood with each beat and has a high level of CRF.

## What Are the Measures of Aerobic Fitness?

Cardiorespiratory fitness values are expressed in the following ways: the number of liters of oxygen used by the body per minute (liters per minute), the number of milliliters of oxygen used per kilogram of body weight per minute (ml/[kg × min]), and METs. One MET describes the amount of oxygen used by the body at rest and is equal to 3.5 ml/[kg × min]. If you have the ability to use 35 ml/[kg × min] during maximal exercise, you are said to have a CRF equal to 10 METs ($35 \div 3.5 = 10$). Aerobic training programs increase the heart's ability to pump blood, so it is no surprise that CRF increases as a result of such programs. As Figure 6.1 shows, most tests used to evaluate CRF use dynamic activities, those involving the large muscle groups in the legs (usually walking, running, stepping, or cycling). The following sections suggest how you should approach such tests, what information is obtained, and how to interpret it.

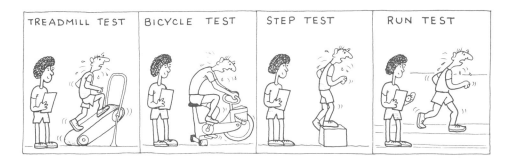

**Figure 6.1** How to analyze cardiorespiratory function.

## What Is a Good Sequence for Testing and Activities?

Figure 6.2 shows the steps involved in evaluating CRF. Begin your testing by participating in the screening process outlined in chapter 3. The guidelines presented in that chapter will help you decide when to take fitness tests and participate in fitness activities. If you have no major medical problems, you can participate in the following types of tests. Generally, the testing process begins with obtaining a series of resting measurements. These could include a blood sample, heart rate, blood pressure, an electrocardiogram (ECG), pulmonary measures to evaluate lung function, and, of course, body fatness. The number and types of measurements will depend on your age, apparent health status, and the facility (if any) involved in your fitness program. Clearly, if you are exercising on your own, it is less likely that sophisticated measurements will be obtained prior to the fitness tests. If you have known medical problems or are at high risk, you should have a physical examination prior to taking a fitness test or starting an exercise program.

If the resting measurements indicate that you can take a fitness test, we recommend a *submaximal* fitness test. Submaximal tests *do not* require you to exercise to your maximum effort, and they reduce the chance that you will have sore muscles the next day. Heart rate and blood pressure are usually measured, and the test is stopped at 70 to 85% of estimated maximal heart rate. The results provide good information related to your CRF, and the test is a sensitive indicator of how you improve over time. In some testing centers an ECG is also measured, depending on the person being tested and the personnel involved. If the measurements are normal, you can now start a fitness program; if not, you may be referred for additional tests or procedures.

In some testing centers the submaximal test is continued past this point, and you may be asked to exercise to maximum. This is more likely in a clinical setting, where using this kind of maximal test increases the chance of finding any abnormalities. However, in some maximal tests no measurements are

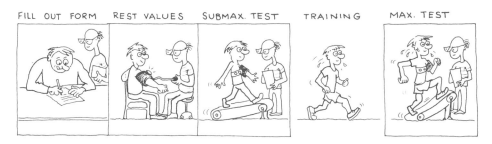

**Figure 6.2** Sequence of testing.

made other than the time to run a given distance. This type of maximal test is *not* recommended at the start of a fitness program.

## What Tests Can I Use?

A variety of field tests can be used to obtain an estimate of CRF. They are called "field tests" because they require very little equipment, can be done just about anywhere, and use the simple activities of walking and running. Because these tests require you to walk or run as fast as you can over a set distance, they are *not* recommended at the start of an exercise program. Instead, we recommend that you begin with the graduated walking and/or jogging programs outlined in chapter 12 before taking these tests. The graduated nature of the fitness program will allow you to start at a low, safe level of activity and gradually improve. It is then appropriate for you to take a test and see how fit you are.

Field tests rely on the observation that for a person to be able to walk or run at high speeds over long distances the heart must pump great volumes of oxygen to the muscles. Therefore, the average speed you maintain in these walk and run tests gives an estimate of your CRF. The higher your CRF score, the greater the capacity of the heart to transport oxygen.

### Walk Test

The one-mile walk test was recently developed as a CRF test for adults, especially older adults. The test should be done on a measured track or other flat surface so that the distance of one mile is clearly identified. For example, four laps on an outdoor running track is usually equal to one mile. If you use an indoor track, mall, or gymnasium, check with someone to make sure of the distance. Stretch out and do some slow walking to warm up. The idea for the test is simply to walk as fast as you can for the one-mile distance (do not run or jog). Use a stopwatch to record your time in minutes and seconds. In addition, at the end of the walk, stop and immediately take your heart rate for 10 seconds to obtain an estimate of the heart rate associated with the walk. The time of the walk and your heart rate value are used to predict your CRF in Table 6.1 (data used to generate table are from Kline et al., 1987). To use Table 6.1, find the section of the table pertaining to your sex and age, then read across the top until you find the time (to the nearest minute) it took you to walk a mile. Look down that column until it intersects with your postexercise heart rate (listed in the far left column). The number where your mile time and postexercise heart rate meet is your CRF value in terms of oxygen used per kilogram of body weight per minute. You can evaluate your aerobic fitness by using that number to compare with the standards presented in Table 6.2. For example, a 25-year-old man who walks the mile in 20 minutes and has a postexercise heart rate of 140 has an estimated maximal oxygen uptake of 29.8 ml/[kg × min]. His maximal oxygen uptake is "borderline," indicating the need for improvement.

### Jog/Run Test

One of the most common CRF field tests is the 12-minute or 1.5-mile run popularized by Dr. Kenneth Cooper. This test is very much like the walk test just described: Jog or run as fast as you can for 12 minutes or for 1.5 miles.

**Table 6.1** (Continued)

| Heart rate | Min/mile | | | | | | | | | | |
|---|---|---|---|---|---|---|---|---|---|---|---|
| | 10 | 11 | 12 | 13 | 14 | 15 | 16 | 17 | 18 | 19 | 20 |
| | | | | | Women (60-69) | | | | | | |
| 120 | 46.6 | 43.3 | 40.0 | 36.8 | 33.5 | 30.2 | 27.0 | 23.7 | 20.5 | 17.2 | 13.9 |
| 130 | 45.0 | 41.7 | 38.5 | 35.2 | 31.9 | 28.7 | 25.4 | 22.2 | 18.9 | 15.6 | 12.4 |
| 140 | 43.4 | 40.2 | 36.9 | 33.6 | 30.4 | 27.1 | 23.8 | 20.6 | 17.3 | 14.1 | 10.8 |
| 150 | 41.9 | 38.6 | 35.3 | 32.1 | 28.8 | 25.5 | 22.3 | 19.0 | 15.8 | 12.5 | 9.2 |
| 160 | 40.3 | 37.0 | 33.8 | 30.5 | 27.2 | 24.0 | 20.7 | 17.5 | 14.2 | 10.9 | 7.7 |

*Note.* Calculations assume 170 lb for men and 125 lb for women. For each 15 lb beyond these values, subtract 1 ml. Adapted from Kline et al. (1987).

Your average running speed is dependent on the ability of your heart and lungs to transport oxygen to the working muscles. This test makes use of this observation, and the CRF score is dependent on the speed you can maintain over the distance. Find a measured track as above, and run as far as you can in 12 minutes, or run 1.5 miles for time. Table 6.2 lists values for CRF as *good*, *adequate*, *borderline*, and *needs extra work*. The table takes age and sex into consideration. For example, a 40-year-old woman who runs 1.5 miles in 14 minutes and 15 seconds (14:15) rates between *adequate* and *good*. This time of 14:15 corresponds to a CRF value of about 35 to 40 ml/[kg × min]. We recommend that you try to achieve and maintain the *good* value for your age group; if you are not at that level, however, plan on making small and systematic progress toward that goal using the walking and jogging programs in chapter 12.

## What Are Graded Exercise Tests?

The field tests already mentioned are "all-out" tests in that you are asked to walk or run as fast as you can. It has become quite common for fitness centers to offer a submaximal test of CRF that does not require an all-out effort. In this test you might walk on a treadmill, step up and down on a bench, or ride a stationary bicycle (cycle ergometer) through a series of progressively more difficult stages until you reach a predetermined end point. Most of these tests are stopped when your heart rate reaches 70 to 85% of your age-adjusted estimate of maximal heart rate, which is calculated by subtracting your age from 220 (220 − age). Typically, heart rate, blood pressure, and an estimate of your subjective effort are obtained at each stage of the test. The most common index of effort is the Rating of Perceived Exertion (RPE) shown in Table 6.3 on page 54. In this scale, higher scores reflect more intense perception of effort; for example, the expression "very, very hard" indicates near-maximal work.

### How Is Heart Rate Used?

Figure 6.3 on page 55 shows how some of this information is used. The heart rate data were collected during a submaximal treadmill test of a 37-year-old

**Table 6.2**
**Standards for Maximal Oxygen Uptake and Endurance Runs**

| Age[a] | $\dot{V}O_2$ max (ml/[kg × min]) | 1.5-mile run (min:s) | 12-min run (miles) |
|---|---|---|---|
| | Men | | |
| | Good | | |
| 15-30 | > 45 | < 10 | > 1.7 |
| 35-50 | > 40 | < 11:30 | > 1.5 |
| 55-70 | > 35 | < 14 | > 1.3 |
| | Adequate for most activities | | |
| 15-30 | 40 | 11:50 | 1.5 |
| 35-50 | 35 | 13 | 1.4 |
| 55-70 | 30 | 15:30 | 1.3 |
| | Borderline | | |
| 15-30 | 35 | 13 | 1.4 |
| 35-50 | 30 | 14:30 | 1.3 |
| 55-70 | 25 | 17 | 1.2 |
| | Needs extra work on CRF | | |
| 15-30 | < 30 | > 15 | < 1.3 |
| 35-50 | < 25 | > 16:30 | < 1.2 |
| 55-70 | < 20 | > 19 | < 1.0 |
| | Women[b] | | |
| | Good | | |
| 15-30 | > 40 | < 12 | > 1.5 |
| 35-50 | > 35 | < 13:30 | > 1.4 |
| 55-70 | > 30 | < 16 | > 1.2 |
| | Adequate for most activities | | |
| 15-30 | 35 | 13:30 | 1.4 |
| 35-50 | 30 | 15 | 1.3 |
| 55-70 | 25 | 17:30 | 1.1 |
| | Borderline | | |
| 15-30 | 30 | 15 | 1.3 |
| 35-50 | 25 | 16:30 | 1.2 |
| 55-70 | 20 | 19 | 1.0 |
| | Needs extra work on CRF | | |
| 15-30 | < 25 | > 17 | < 1.2 |
| 35-50 | < 20 | > 18:30 | < 1.1 |
| 55-70 | < 15 | > 21 | < 0.9 |

*Note.* These standards are for fitness programs. People wanting to do well in endurance performance need higher levels. For those at the *Good* level, the emphasis is on maintaining this level the rest of their lives. For those in the lower levels, emphasis is on setting and reaching realistic goals. Adapted from Howley and Franks (1986).

[a]Aerobic fitness declines with age. [b]Women have lower standards because they have a larger amount of essential fat.

**Table 6.3**
**Rating of Perceived Exertion**

| Rating | Description |
| --- | --- |
| | Original scale |
| 6 | |
| 7 | Very, very light |
| 8 | |
| 9 | Very light |
| 10 | |
| 11 | Fairly light |
| 12 | |
| 13 | Somewhat hard |
| 14 | |
| 15 | Hard |
| 16 | |
| 17 | Very hard |
| 18 | |
| 19 | Very, very hard |
| 20 | |
| | Revised scale |
| 0 | Nothing |
| 0.5 | Very, very light (just noticeable) |
| 1.0 | Very light |
| 2 | Light (weak) |
| 3 | Moderate |
| 4 | Somewhat hard |
| 5 | Heavy (strong) |
| 6 | |
| 7 | Very heavy |
| 8 | |
| 9 | |
| 10 | Very, very heavy (almost max) |

*Note.* From G.A.V. Borg, "Psychological Bases of Physical Exertion," Medicine and Science in Sports and Exercise, **14**(5), 377-381, © by American College of Sports Medicine, 1982.

man whose estimated maximal heart rate was 183 beats per minute (220 − 37 = 183). The test used a walking speed of 3 miles per hour, and the grade (elevation) of the treadmill was increased 2.5% after each 2 minutes of the test. The man's heart rate was plotted against the grade, and a solid line was drawn through the points up to the last heart rate value measured in the test (85% of maximal heart rate). At this stage the test was still submaximal. A dashed line was then drawn along the same path up to the man's estimated maximal heart rate. At this point another line was "dropped" to the lower axis of the graph to indicate what the person's maximal work level would have been had he reached this stage of the test. The lower axis of the graph indicates the percent grade of the treadmill and the MET value equal to that grade. In this way a *submaximal* test can be used to estimate *maximal* aerobic fitness.

How does this submaximal test show changes in CRF that have resulted from a training program? One of the most consistent results of endurance training is that heart rate response is lower at any given stage of the test. So

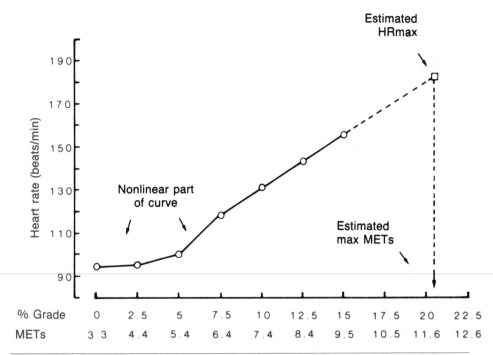

**Figure 6.3** Estimating maximal aerobic power. *Note.* From Howley and Franks (1986).

if your heart rate response is 150 beats per minute at 15% grade before training, the value for the same work level may be only 130 beats per minute after training. You may therefore need to complete another stage or two of the test before you reach your 85% of maximal heart rate cutoff.

## How Are Blood Pressure Measurements Used?

Your blood pressure is monitored during a graded exercise test to provide additional information about how you adjust to increasing work rates. Blood pressure is given as two separate scores. The first and higher number is called *systolic blood pressure* and represents the highest pressure during a heartbeat; the second and lower number is *diastolic blood pressure* and is the pressure in the cardiovascular system when the heart is at rest. During a graded exercise test systolic pressure usually increases with each stage, while diastolic pressure decreases slightly or remains the same. If you do not respond in this manner, or if your systolic value becomes extremely high, the test is stopped before you achieve your 85% of maximal heart rate cutoff point.

## What Is the Rating of Perceived Exertion?

The RPE usually increases with each stage of a graded exercise test and is used as an indication of how close you may be to your maximum work load. This is a good measure to obtain because your estimated maximal heart rate value is only an *estimate* and may actually be too high or too low. Like any estimate, the formula 220 – age cannot predict each individual's maximal heart rate with exact precision (you have to do a maximal test to find your actual maximal heart rate value). Because the estimate of maximal heart rate may be as much as 20 beats per minute too high or too low, the RPE score gives another indication of when you are reaching your personal end point.

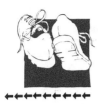

## Summary

This chapter helped you to evaluate your cardiorespiratory fitness level. You can use a walking test combined with heart rate measurement to estimate your maximal aerobic power. If you are tested in a fitness program, this chapter described how heart rate, blood pressure, and perceived exertion might be used in a graded exercise test. It is important to emphasize that resting, submaximal tests, *and a beginning conditioning program* should all precede all-out field tests. If you are beginning a fitness program on your own, you should *not* use a running test to determine your cardiorespiratory fitness level until after you have successfully completed a beginning fitness program (e.g., the walking and jogging programs presented in chapter 12).

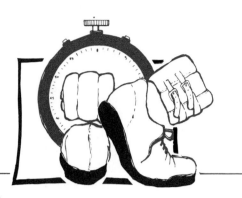

## Chapter
## 7

# How Can I Increase Muscular Strength and Endurance?

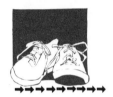

**What Is Muscular Strength?**

**What Is Muscular Endurance?**

**What Exercises Improve Strength and Endurance?**

Muscular strength describes the *maximum force* that can be generated by a muscle. A person with a great deal of strength can lift very heavy weights. Strength is dependent on the size of the muscle and the ability to "recruit" available muscle fibers, which is related to the individual's level of arousal. In contrast, muscular endurance describes the ability of a muscle to make repeated contractions against a *less-than-maximal* load. An individual who can lift a weight many times before experiencing fatigue has a high level of muscular endurance. Do you need muscular strength and endurance to achieve a high level of health-related fitness?

In general, we believe that both muscular strength and muscular endurance should be developed and maintained at levels that make the activities of daily living comfortable. Some people need higher levels than others because of their occupational or recreational pursuits. However, it is difficult to pinpoint some absolute quantity of muscular strength and endurance needed to minimize the degenerative diseases associated with inactivity. The focus of attention in health-related fitness programs, as we have discussed in previous chapters, is on cardiorespiratory fitness and an appropriate level of body fatness. An exception to this statement is the recognized need for abdominal muscle strength and endurance to help prevent or relieve low back pain (see chapter 9).

## How Is Muscular Strength Measured?

How strong are you? Your answer depends, in part, on the type of strength test you take. Strength is measured with *isometric*, *isokinetic*, and *isotonic* tests.

*Isometric strength* is measured with instruments such as the *grip dynamometer*, which measures the force of your grip, or the *cable tensiometer*, which can measure the strength of most muscle groups. In an isometric contraction the muscle does not shorten (isometric = constant length) even though the person is exerting maximal force. Isometric strength varies with the angle of the joint and does not provide a measure of strength throughout the normal range of motion of a joint.

*Isokinetic strength* is measured with a special machine that controls the speed at which you can move a joint through its range of motion. A limb, such as the lower leg, is attached to a lever arm that controls how fast the limb moves. When a muscle contracts with as much force as possible to move the limb, sensors in the machine monitor strength throughout the range of motion. These machines are expensive and can usually be found in physical therapy and athletic training facilities.

*Isotonic strength* is the type of strength measure with which you are most familiar. Strength is simply measured as the heaviest weight lifted through a normal range of motion. For example, Figure 7.1 shows the arm-curl test being used to measure the strength of the bicep muscle (located on the front of the upper arm). This maximal strength value is called your One Repetition Maximum, or *1RM*.

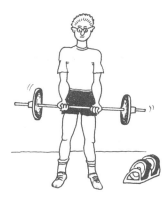

**Figure 7.1** Isotonic strength test.

## How Is Muscular Endurance Measured?

Muscular endurance is typically measured by counting the number of lifts you can do with a fixed weight. This is sometimes called *absolute muscular endurance*, as the weight that is lifted is a fixed (absolute) quantity. This approach can be used to show progress over time. A person might have been able to do only five arm curls with a 25-pound weight prior to a training program but increased that number to 20 after the program.

Another approach is to measure *relative muscular endurance*, which shows how many times you can lift a weight that is a certain percent (e.g., 70%) of your 1RM. Because the 1RM (maximal strength) will change during a training program, this approach allows you to see how your muscular endurance changes as your strength increases. For example, at the beginning of a training program your 1RM might be 60 pounds for an arm curl and you might lift 42 pounds (70% of 60 pounds) 10 times. At the end of the training program your 1RM might be 80 pounds and you might lift 56 pounds (70% of 80 pounds) only six times. In this case muscular strength increased faster than muscular endurance.

## What Principles Should I Follow in Training?

The principles of *overload* and *specificity*, which we will discuss more extensively in chapter 11, apply rather well to training programs for muscular strength and endurance. The overload principle states that to make improvements, a muscle must lift a heavier weight than that to which it is accustomed. As your muscle adapts to that new heavier load you must overload the muscle again if you desire additional strength gains (see Figure 7.2).

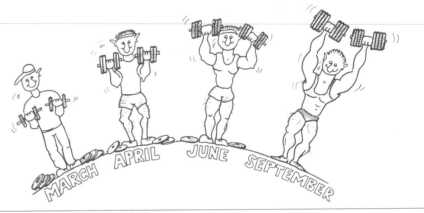

**Figure 7.2** The overload principle.

The principle of specificity states that the type of adaptation that occurs is related to the type of exercise used. It is best illustrated by comparisons between gains in muscular strength and gains in muscular endurance. If a person lifts heavy weights the primary change is an increase in the *size* of the muscle cell, a process called *hypertrophy*. This increase in muscle size is associated with the increase in muscle strength. On the other hand, if a person does many repetitions with lighter weights (e.g., 50% of 1RM), the primary changes in muscle are found in the energy-producing parts, called mitochondria, and in the number of capillaries that bring oxygen to the muscle cell. Muscle size does not increase very much with endurance exercise. Though in general the effects of training are specific to the type of exercise performed, there is some overlap in the areas of strength and endurance because a person cannot completely isolate one from the other.

## What Training Programs Develop Muscular Strength and Endurance?

*Progressive Resistance Exercise (PRE)* is a general term that describes a method to progressively and systematically overload a muscle group. A PRE program specifies both the weight (*load*) lifted and the maximum number of repetitions the load is lifted (*RM*). The term *set* describes the number of repetitions done before a rest. For example, if you were to do three sets of a

10-RM routine, you would choose a weight (see below) you can lift a maximum of 10 times (10 RM), and do the following:

1. Lift weight 10 times; rest.
2. Lift weight 10 times; rest.
3. Lift weight 10 times; rest.

For optimal gains in muscular *strength*, follow a 4 to 8 RM routine (choose a weight you can lift a maximum of 4 to 8 times), and do three sets. When you can lift the weight more than eight times in each of three sets, increase the weight (the overload principle). In this way you are progressively increasing the load against which the muscle must work. For optimal gains in muscular *endurance* do three sets of a 10- to 25-RM routine. High repetitions with lighter weights result in specific muscular endurance adaptations. Weight training, like aerobics, is done on an *every-other-day* basis.

## Weight Training

The first question to ask in a weight training program is: How much weight should I start with? Two general guidelines follow:

1. For exercises with the arms start your PRE program with a weight equal to one fourth to one third of your body weight. If you weigh 180 pounds start with 45 (1/4 of 180) to 60 (1/3 of 180) pounds.
2. For exercises with the legs start your PRE program with a weight equal to one half to two thirds of your body weight. If you weigh 180 pounds start with 90 (1/2 of 180) to 120 (2/3 of 180) pounds.

Table 7.1 provides a summary of starting weights for people of different body weights.

**Table 7.1**
**Starting Weights (in Pounds) for Weight Training for Arms and Legs**

| Body weight (lb) | Arms | Legs |
|---|---|---|
| 100 | 25-33 | 50- 67 |
| 120 | 30-40 | 60- 80 |
| 140 | 35-46 | 70- 93 |
| 160 | 40-53 | 80-107 |
| 180 | 45-60 | 90-120 |
| 200 | 50-66 | 100-133 |

Remember, in choosing a starting point in your PRE program, *it is better to do too little rather than too much.*

The following are selected weight training activities that provide for an increase in muscular strength and endurance (see Figures 7.3a to 7.3f).

## Muscular Strength and Endurance Without Weights

Generally, if your training program includes running, cycling, or dancing you are providing enough stimulus to maintain an adequate level of muscular strength and endurance in your leg muscles. However, those activities do little

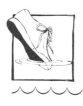

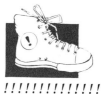

!!!!!!!!!!!!!!

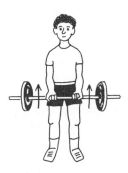

**Figure 7.3a** *Arm Curl.* With arms extended, hold the barbell with an underhand grip. While keeping the elbows close to the sides, flex the forearms and raise the barbell to the chest, lower to the starting position. Suggested beginning load: ¼ to ⅓ of body weight.

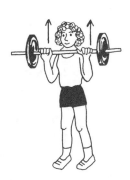

**Figure 7.3b** *Overhead Press.* Hold the barbell at chest level with an overhand grip. Push the bar straight up to full extension and then lower to the starting position. Do not hyperextend the back. Suggested beginning load: ¼ to ⅓ of body weight.

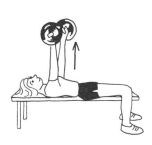

**Figure 7.3c** *Bench Press.* Hold barbell above chest with hands slightly wider than shoulder width. Lower barbell to chest and push back to starting position. Suggested starting load: ¼ to ⅓ of body weight.

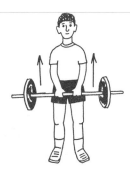

**Figure 7.3d** *Upright Rowing.* Hold barbell with an overhand grip with hands one to two inches apart. Keep elbows above the bar while raising it to shoulder position. Suggested beginning load: ¼ to ⅓ of body weight.

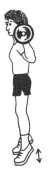

**Figure 7.3e** *Heel Lifts.* With barbell behind shoulder at the back of the neck, raise upward on toes and then slowly return the heels to the floor. Suggested beginning load: ½ to ⅔ of body weight.

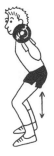

**Figure 7.3f** *Half Squats.* With barbell behind shoulders at the back of the neck, gradually lower body to a semi-squat position. Keep back straight. Suggested beginning load: ½ to ⅔ of body weight.

**Figure 7.3a-f** Weight training program for developing strength.

for the muscular strength of your arms, shoulders, or trunk. One of the most common ways to increase muscular strength and endurance for those muscle groups is to do exercises in which your own body acts as the weight or resistance against which you work. The following activities focus attention on strength and endurance development in the arms and shoulders.

Figure 7.4 shows three forms of push-ups that vary in difficulty and can be done anywhere: the push-away, the bent-knee push-up, and the regular push-up. Start with the push-away until you can comfortably do three sets of 10 in one workout. When you accomplish this goal, try the bent knee push-up, starting with two sets of 5 and increasing until you can do two sets of 10 in a single workout. Finally, shift to the regular push-up, doing two sets of 5, and gradually work up to two sets of 10. When you have accomplished this goal, continue to do the two sets of 10 in each workout.

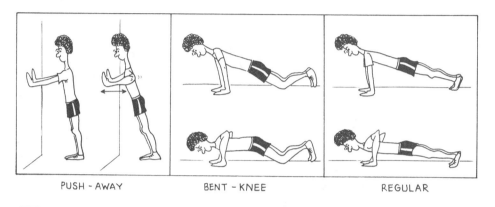

PUSH - AWAY          BENT - KNEE          REGULAR

**Figure 7.4** Different types of push-ups.

Figure 7.5 shows two types of pull-ups that can be used to gain strength and endurance. The standard pull-up is harder to do because the entire body weight must be pulled up. It is not uncommon for some people to be unable to do a single pull-up. On the other hand, body weight is partially supported in the modified pull-up, making it easier to do. Start with two or three modi-

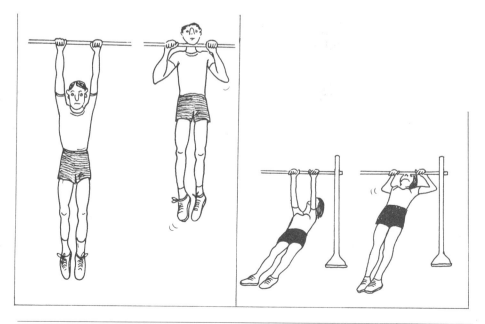

**Figure 7.5** Two types of pull-ups—standard (left) and modified (right).

fied pull-ups, adding some when you are able, gradually working up to doing 25 to 35.

Another exercise that you can use to strengthen your upper body is the "dip" shown in Figure 7.6. Two versions are presented, with the weight-supported version being the easier of the two.

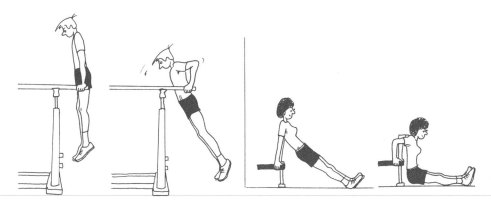

**Figure 7.6** Two versions of the dip—standard (left) and weight-supported (right).

## Summary

Muscular strength is a measure of the maximal force a muscle can generate. Muscular endurance is a measure of the muscle's ability to repeatedly lift a less-than-maximal load. In training programs for strength gains, choose a weight that can be lifted four to eight times and do three sets. For endurance, choose a weight that can be lifted 10 to 25 times and do three sets. The starting weight for arm exercises is one fourth to one third of body weight; for leg exercises, one half to two thirds of body weight. It is better to do too little rather than too much. Use simple push-ups, pull-ups, and dips to promote strength and endurance.

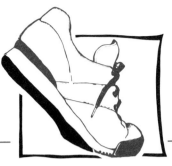

*Chapter*
**8**

# How Can I Increase My Flexibility Through Stretching?

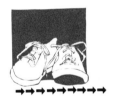

> **What Is Flexibility?**
> **What Exercises Improve Flexibility?**
> **What Exercises Should I Avoid?**

Flexibility is a measure of a joint's ability to move through a normal range of motion. For example, starting with your arms held straight at your sides, can you raise your arms out to the side and up until your hands touch high over your head? If you can, you have a normal range of motion (flexibility) in your shoulder joints.

Each joint has a limited range of motion, depending on the joint. It is important to maintain the flexibility of each joint so that normal everyday tasks can be completed without undue strain. Lack of flexibility can be related to medical problems, with low back pain being one example (see chapter 9).

## What Causes a Lack of Flexibility?

Flexibility, like any trait, is limited by our genetic endowment. It is clear, however, that regular use is necessary to develop and maintain that endowment. For example, when a cast is removed from someone who had a broken bone at the elbow joint, that person's initial attempts to move the joint through its normal range of motion are usually not very successful and are perceived as painful. What causes the lack of flexibility at the elbow joint? While the arm is immobilized in the cast, fibrous connective tissue, or "adhesions," begin to cling to the tendons, ligaments, and bones in the joint, reducing its range of motion. In addition, due to the fact that the cast holds the arm at a fixed angle, the upper arm muscles become shortened and do not allow the arm to straighten when the cast is removed. Flexibility, then, is affected by both the condition of the connective tissues at the joint and the ability of the muscle to

### Reach Back

Stand with feet shoulder-width apart and hold your arms out to the sides with thumbs pointing down. *Slowly* move both arms back until tension is felt. Hold for 10 to 30 seconds and relax.

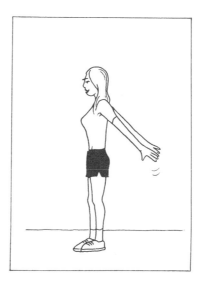

**Figure 8.3**   Reach back.

### Arm Circles

Stand with feet shoulder-width apart and hold arms straight out to the side. Start moving your arms *slowly* in small circles, which gradually become larger and larger circles. Come back to the starting position and reverse the direction of your arm swing.

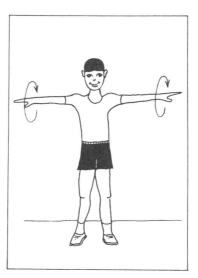

**Figure 8.4**   Arm circles.

## TRUNK

### *Side Bend*

Standing with feet shoulder-width apart, raise your right arm over your head with the elbow slightly bent. *Slowly* bend to the left side until slight tension is felt. Hold for 10 to 30 seconds and relax. Repeat for other side.

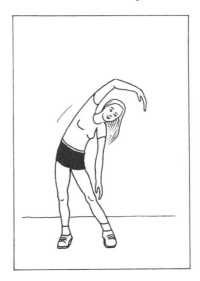

**Figure 8.5**  Side bend.

### *Sit and Twist*

Sit on a mat with your left leg straight in front of you. Bend your right leg and cross it over your left leg so that your right foot is alongside your left knee. Bring your left elbow across your body and place it on the outside of your right thigh near the knee. *Slowly* twist your body as you look over your right shoulder. Your left elbow should be exerting pressure against your right thigh. Hold the stretch for 10 to 30 seconds, relax, and repeat for the other side.

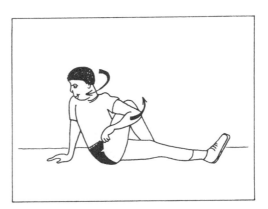

**Figure 8.6**  Sit and twist.

### Knee to Chest

Lie on your back on a mat with your legs straight. Bend your right knee and bring it up toward your chest. Grasp the underside of your thigh and *slowly* pull your thigh to your chest. Hold for 10 to 30 seconds. Release, and repeat with the left leg.

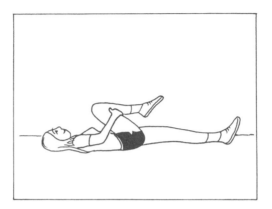

**Figure 8.7** Knee to chest.

## GROIN

### Groin Stretch

Sit on a mat with your knees bent. Put the soles of your feet (or shoes) together and hold onto your ankles. Place your elbows on the inner side of your knees and *slowly* apply downward pressure until you feel tension. Hold for 10 to 30 seconds and repeat.

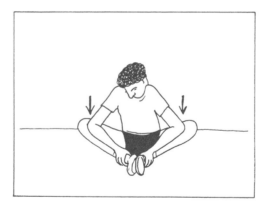

**Figure 8.8** Groin stretch.

## LEGS

### *Quad Stretch*

Stand with your right hand against a wall, a post, or another person. Bend your right knee while moving your foot upward and backward. Use your left hand to grasp the foot and *slowly* bring it up and across your body until you feel tension on the front side of the thigh. Hold for 10 to 30 seconds and repeat for the left leg.

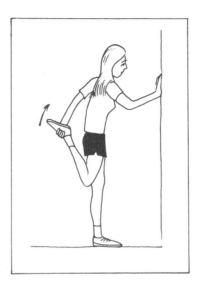

**Figure 8.9** Quad stretch.

### *Hamstring Stretch*

While standing, raise your right foot onto a table, bench, or chair so that your leg is almost parallel to the floor. *Slowly* move your hands along your right leg toward your ankle until you feel tension on the underside of the thigh. Hold the tension for 10 to 30 seconds and relax. Repeat for the other leg.

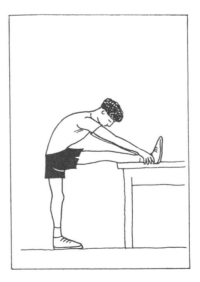

**Figure 8.10** Hamstring stretch.

### Achilles Stretch

Stand facing a wall with your right foot close to the wall and your right knee bent. With your left leg straight, *slowly* lean toward the wall, *keeping your left heel flat on the ground.* Hold for 10 to 30 seconds and relax. Repeat for the right leg.

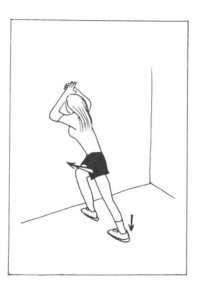

**Figure 8.11**  Achilles stretch.

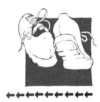

## Summary

Flexibility is a measure of how well a joint can move through its normal range of motion. Flexibility is limited by both the connective tissues at the joint and the muscles that are responsible for moving the joint. Stretching exercises increase a joint's flexibility by acting on both types of tissue, and flexibility is lost when those specific exercises are not done on a regular basis. Include stretching exercises as a regular part of your warm-up and cool-down.

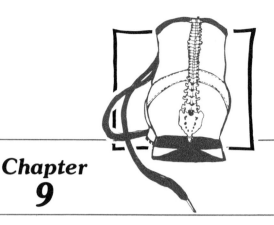

**Chapter
9**

# How Can I Prevent
# Low Back Problems?

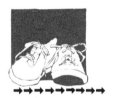

**What Causes Back Problems?**

**What Can I Do to Prevent Back Problems?**

**What Tests Can Help Me Measure Progress in Prevention?**

Has your back ever hurt? If it has, you can understand why low back pain is one of the most common complaints among adults in the United States. Low back problems account for more lost person hours than any other type of occupational injury and are the most frequent cause of activity limitation in U.S. citizens under age 45. If you have never had low back problems, be grateful and include some daily preventive exercises to help reduce the chance that the problem will occur.

## What Causes Low Back Pain?

Many factors are related to low back problems, including structural abnormalities, some diseases, accidents, inappropriate lifting, poor posture, lack of warm-up prior to vigorous activity, lack of abdominal strength and endurance, lack of flexibility in the back and legs, and inability to cope with stressors.

### Structural Abnormalities

A very *small* percentage of low back problems are caused by anatomical problems (e.g., a deformed spine, one leg longer than the other). These conditions may be altered by some structural device or may require surgery.

Many exercises that have been used in the past to strengthen the abdominal area actually appear to make the problem worse rather than better. For example, *avoid* the following: straight-leg sit-ups, sit-ups performed with someone holding your feet, timed sit-ups, and double-leg raises (see Figure 9.3).

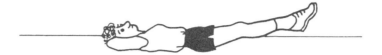

**Figure 9.3** *Exercise to avoid*—double leg raises.

The best type of exercise for the abdominal region is a slow curl-up with knees bent and feet flat but not held (see Figure 9.4). The curl-up is the first part of a sit-up, but instead of coming all the way up to a sitting position, you stop at what is called the "sticking point." This is the point in the sit-up where it would require additional effort—more muscle involvement—to come all the way up. Your abdominal muscles do the work during the curl-up stage, but you have to use additional muscles to go from the sticking point all the way up to a sit-up. Since we are most interested in working the abdominal muscles, a curl-up is the recommended exercise. Do these curl-ups slowly and increase the number done gradually over time until you can do a total of 30 to 40 each day.

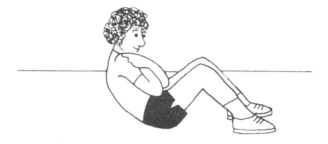

**Figure 9.4** Curl-up.

## Flexibility

Chapter 8 dealt with total body flexibility. An important component related to low back problems is the amount of flexibility you have in the low back and upper legs. The muscles that move the hips in different directions are associated with low back pain. Either lack of flexibility or lack of strength and endurance in this region can result in back problems. One way to deal with this problem is to do static stretching, which involves slowly lengthening the muscle(s) to a point of slight discomfort; when you reach this point hold the position for 10 to 30 seconds, with one or two repeats. Try that with each of the exercises in chapter 8. Progressively increasing the range of motion results in improved flexibility.

Most low back stretches involve flexion of the back (moving forward). Some extension (moving backward) and slight hyperextension is recommended for most people. If you already have a back problem or you experience pain with hyperextension, seek medical advice. For most folks, some hyperextension is recommended (e.g., see figure 9.5), but *don't* go as far as you can backward in the hyperextension.

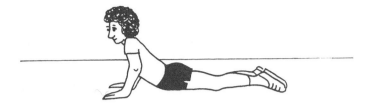

**Figure 9.5** Back hyperextension exercise.

Whenever possible, do these exercises sitting or lying rather than standing. For example, it is better to sit with one leg out and the other flexed and stretch toward one's toes on the extended leg (see Figure 9.6) than to do a standing toe touch (Figure 9.7).

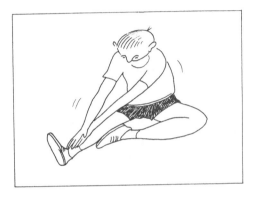

**Figure 9.6** Modified hurdler's stretch.

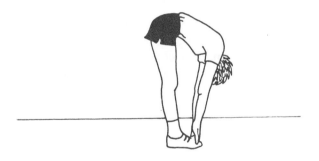

**Figure 9.7** *Exercise to avoid*—standing toe touch.

### Coping With Stressors

Although inability to cope with stressors will not cause back problems if your back is strong, it does cause problems in persons already at risk for back problems. Suggestions for coping with stressors are included in chapter 10.

## How Can I Test My Progress?

You can take tests for muscular strength, endurance, and flexibility in the midtrunk region periodically so you can see how much progress you are making.

## Abdominal Strength and Endurance

Chapter 7 included some tests for overall muscular strength and endurance. Because abdominal strength and endurance play an important role in the prevention of low back pain, a modified curl-up test is presented in this chapter; a low score on this test may indicate a high risk for low back problems.

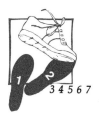

### Curl-Up Test

Steps in taking the curl-up test are listed in Table 9.1.

**Table 9.1**
**Curl-Ups**

| Step | Activity |
| --- | --- |
| 1 | Lie on back with knees at about 90° angle, arms extended with fingers on thighs. |
| 2 | Slowly curl up until fingertips touch knees, then back down (about one curl every 3 seconds). |
| 3 | Count number of curls (i.e., fingertips to knees and head back down). |
| 4 | Do as many as can be done without stopping up to maximal of 35. |
| 5 | Record number of curl-ups on score sheet or card. |

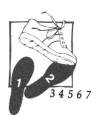

### Flexibility

A test commonly used by fitness instructors is the sit-and-reach test, where you sit with your feet against a box and see how far you can stretch your arms in front of you. A simple test to estimate your flexibility in the posterior thigh (i.e., hamstrings) and low back area uses the stretch found in Figure 9.6. The steps involved in taking this flexibility test are listed in Table 9.2.

**Table 9.2**
**Flexibility Test**

| Step | Activity |
| --- | --- |
| 1 | Warm up with static stretches prior to this test. |
| 2 | Sit with one leg extended and the other one bent so that the bottom of the foot on the second leg is against the inside of the knee of the extended leg (see Figure 9.6). |
| 3 | Place one hand on top of the other and extend arms toward the toes of the extended leg. |
| 4 | Keep knee of extended leg straight. |
| 5 | Reach forward *slowly* as far as possible four times. |
| 6 | If you can reach your foot or beyond, that is good. |
| 7 | If you cannot reach your foot, estimate how far you are from your toes (retest periodically to determine your improvement). |
| 8 | Repeat for the other side. |

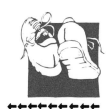

## Summary

Low back problems are caused by a number of factors, including structural abnormalities, disease, accidents, poor posture or lifting mechanics, lack of warm-up before exercise, and lack of flexibility and muscular strength and endurance in the midtrunk area. Many of these problems can be prevented by using appropriate lifting techniques and good posture; warming up before exercise; increasing midtrunk strength/endurance and flexibility; and learning to cope with stress. Use the suggestions in this chapter for lifting, posture, and ways to increase midtrunk flexibility and strength/endurance to greatly lower your risk of low back problems in the future.

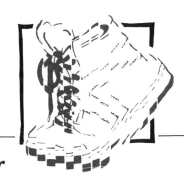

# Chapter
# *10*

# *How Can I Cope With Stress?*

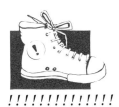

| **How Is Stress Related to Health?** |
| **Can Physical Activity Reduce Stress?** |
| **How Can I Cope With Stressors?** |

Cardiovascular function, relative leanness, and low back function have been accepted as physical fitness components. Physical fitness also assumes sufficient levels of flexibility and muscular strength and endurance to be able to do daily tasks efficiently.

Though we acknowledge our inability to separate the mental, physical, psychological, social, and spiritual aspects of life, this book has emphasized *physical* fitness. This chapter deals with an area that bridges the psychological and physiological aspects of fitness.

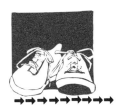

## What Are the Psychological Aspects of Fitness?

The fit person can work and play with vigor and enthusiasm. The healthy life also involves the ability to relax and disregard irrelevant stimuli during quiet times. Vitality and relaxation are both enhanced by physical conditioning.

One of the keys to living the healthy life is balancing arousal and relaxation. People who are always relaxed and easygoing don't accomplish very much. On the other hand, people who have a "get up and go" attitude toward all aspects of life at all times exhibit coronary-prone behavior.

This chapter deals with the idea of balance by describing the relationships among personality, physical activity, stress, and health. It is beyond the scope of the chapter to discuss all psychological aspects of fitness extensively. Pathological traits or behaviors should be referred to health professionals who specialize in treating such problems. Our concern here is with "normal" levels of personality and stress and their implications for fitness programs.

*Motivation.* We are concerned with motives for exercise at two levels. The first level: How can *we* get you to *begin* a fitness program? The public has been educated to realize in general what healthy behaviors are (most people agree that they should exercise on a regular basis). However, there must be convenient programs available that provide personal contact with concerned exercise professionals to complement information about the healthy life. The second level: What will make you *continue* exercise as a part of your lifestyle? Individual attention, realistic goals with periodic evaluation, option for group participation, involvement of spouse and/or important others, contracts, and programs that minimize injury all seem to help people adhere to fitness programs. Whether motivating you to begin or to continue activity, fitness has to achieve priority status (like eating and sleeping) in your life. Any efforts to increase motivation must have that end in sight. Therefore, external, or extrinsic, rewards must be viewed as a temporary means to change behavior; behavior can be maintained over the long haul only with internal, or intrinsic, motivation.

*Play and Goal Orientation.* One of the key elements in achieving an arousal/relaxation balance is to appreciate the balance of work and play. One individual has difficulty taking time just to play and enjoy an activity not directly related to productivity; another has a problem in getting down to business and getting a task done. People who try to pattern their fitness programs after military or athletic models often have a goal orientation without the play. Others who are not discriminating about their selection of activities as long as everyone is having a good time may achieve playfulness without fitness gains. The good fitness program achieves this balance by including activities designed to improve the necessary fitness components as well as a "playful" atmosphere where it is fun to participate.

*State/Trait.* Making the distinction between your "usual" (*trait*) personality characteristics and specific "situational" (*state*) personality characteristics is helpful in dealing with your personality. For example, you may normally be very quiet and introverted, but you become an extrovert during competitive games. You may normally be very relaxed, but you get anxious about exercise. Generally, personality traits do not change very much, or quickly. Understanding your traits can help you deal with yourself on a long-term basis. Personality and emotional states vary with situations and are more susceptible to change. For example, if you are afraid or anxious about a physical activity, ease into the activity and progress in small increments until you are relaxed and unafraid when exercising.

## Stress Continuums

Personality is related to stress in that your *perception* of a stimulus or situation determines to a large extent how stressful it is to you. There is no uniform agreement on definitions of stress terms. For our purposes, a stressor is defined as any stimulus or condition related to an activity that causes physiological arousal beyond what is necessary to accomplish the activity. This excessive arousal is called stress.

There are three major components of stress. A complete description of a stressful event includes the amount by which the stress response exceeds the functional demand, how pleasant it is to the individual, and whether it causes development or deterioration. These components are explained below.

*Functional . . . Severe Stress.* An individual's physiological response to stress at any one time lies on a continuum from what is essential to provide the energy for that task at one end of the continuum to extreme physiological response beyond what is needed at the other end. Table 10.1 illustrates how typical resting and submaximal heart rates include not only the heart rate needed to provide energy for the body, but increased heart rate (stress) due to chronic stressors (e.g., excess fat) and acute stressors (e.g., agitated emotional state).

**Table 10.1**
**Stress Components of Heart Rate**

| Component of heart rate (HR) | Heart rate (beats/min) | | |
| --- | --- | --- | --- |
| | Sitting | Climbing stairs | Running |
| HR needed to do task | 30 | 50 | 100 |
| Additional HR due to chronic stressors | | | |
| Poor aerobic fitness | +15 | +20 | +40 |
| Excess fat | + 5 | +15 | +20 |
| Additional HR due to acute stressors | | | |
| Not relaxed | +10 | + 5 | 0 |
| Emotional state | +15 | +10 | 0 |
| Total heart rate | 75 | 100 | 160 |

*Note.* This HR model shows the contribution of the heart rate necessary to perform various tasks and the additional HR response caused by chronic and acute stressors. The actual HR values will vary with the individual depending on body size, fitness level, and type and severity of stressors. Adapted from Howley and Franks (1986).

*Enjoyable . . . Unpleasant.* Another aspect of stress is how enjoyable you perceive the stressor to be. Attending an exciting concert and taking an examination to qualify for a position may provoke similar stress responses; however, you probably perceive the concert as more enjoyable.

*Development . . . Deterioration.* The third aspect of stress is what happens to you as a result of the stressful experience. This is, of course, the main criterion for determining whether the stressful event was positive or negative. Positive stressors result in a healthier, stronger person. Negative stressors lead to a weaker individual. The end result of stress is somewhat independent of the other two aspects of stress. For example, a very stressful event (i.e., one that causes a large stress response beyond what is essential physically) can result in your being inspired to achieve great things, or it may destroy your initiative. On the other hand, conditions that cause little stress response may lead to steady development or can gradually wear down your desire to excel. In addition, you can grow and develop from stressors that are pleasant (e.g., positive reinforcement) as well as those that are unpleasant (e.g., a deadline to finish a project). Either pleasant or unpleasant stressors may tempt you to escape from confronting important areas of your life.

Therefore be cautious in identifying a specific stressor as healthy or unhealthy based just on the degree of physiological and psychological stress response, or how pleasant you find the situation. A better criterion is to determine whether the experience has led you toward higher levels of mental, social, and/or physical health.

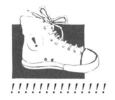

!!!!!!!!!!!!!!!

## How Is Stress Related to Health?

Stress is important to both positive and negative aspects of health. No discussion of the highest quality of life possible nor of serious health problems is complete without including the relevance of stress.

### Positive Stress

We often think of stress as a primarily negative influence on our lives, but it has many positive features.

*Variety.*   Involvement with many stimuli and stressors provides interesting aspects to the full life. You would live a bland existence without stress.

*Development and Growth.*   It is difficult to imagine persons developing, learning, growing, and striving toward their optimal potential without encountering stress.

*Special High Moments.*   One feature of the good life is involvement in special emotional experiences that are remembered forever. It is likely that these peak moments were stressful.

### Negative Stress

Stress is also encountered in any discussion of our society's health problems.

*Secondary Risk Factor.*   Stress is listed as a risk factor for many major health problems—coronary heart disease, hypertension, cancer, ulcers, low back pain, and headaches, for example. Although inability to cope with stress is probably insufficient to cause any of these problems all by itself, stress does seem to exacerbate them. So for some persons, stress results in a heart attack; for others, hypertension, ulcers, low back pain, or headaches.

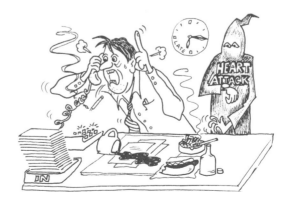

**Figure 10.2**  Negative aspects of stress.

*Susceptibility to Other Stressors.* Inability to cope with one stressor affects the ability to cope with other stressors. All of us have found ourselves getting upset (stressed) over something that normally would not bother us because of stressors in another area of our lives. Two aspects of our inability to cope are our perceptions of and reactions to stressors. Although the positive transfer of our adaptation from one stressor to other stressors is an open question, there is little doubt that there is a negative transfer from an inability to cope in one area leading to problems coping with other areas of life.

## What Role Does Physical Activity Play in Reducing Stress?

Many writers have justified exercise programs partly on the basis that they reduce stress. Although the claims have often exceeded the evidence, there is some support for the statements that stress is reduced as a result of a single period or bout of exercise (acute exercise) as well as over the course of a conditioning program (chronic exercise). Too much exercise, however, can be an additional stressor for people at all levels of fitness. The following illustrations of how exercise can reduce stress assume that you do enough but not too much exercise (see chapter 12).

### Acute Activity

There are three primary ways that single bouts of exercise can reduce stress.

*Distraction.* Exercise (like many other activities) can serve as a temporary distraction from stressors. It is often helpful to step away from a problem, then come back to it later. This technique is healthy as long as exercise doesn't become an escape from the problem. The ultimate reduction of stress must come from coping with the stressor(s). However, one part of your coping strategy can be the distraction of physical activity. Learn to "listen" to your body, to let it give you signals as to when is a good time to step away from a problem and do a fitness workout.

*Control of Situations.* One of the primary concepts in a person's ability to cope with stressors is the perception of personal control. In some cases exercise enhances this feeling of control. For example, increased practice and skill acquisition as a result of an exercise program causes less stress when playing a game in the presence of others. One of the benefits of a postcardiac exercise program is that it reduces the participant's fear that any exertion will cause another heart attack, thus increasing the participant's feelings of control over his or her life.

*Interaction With Others.* A third way that acute exercise may influence stress is by giving you solitary time. For some people one of their daily stressors is constant contact with other people. For example, a working parent spends almost every waking moment in the presence of others—children, spouse, employees, employer, colleagues—who demand time and attention. That person can use a walk or jog program as a time to be alone with his or her thoughts. At the other extreme is a person who has little contact with others during a typical day, with loneliness a potential stressor. Doing activities with other people in an exercise program can aid that person.

- Left arm below elbow
- Right arm below shoulder
- Left arm below shoulder
- Both arms below shoulders
- Chest
- Neck
- Jaw
- Forehead
- Entire head
- Entire body

Extend this last relaxation period—feel the tension leaving your body, and "feel" your breathing.

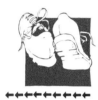

## Summary

This chapter helped you understand what stress is and how you can get its positive benefits while reducing its negative aspects. Stress was defined as excessive arousal beyond what is needed to accomplish a task. Small or large amounts of stress may be either enjoyable or unpleasant. The most important way to evaluate a stressful event is to determine whether it has led to healthy development or deterioration. Ways to maximize the positive elements of stress include exposure to varied stimuli, developing a range of coping abilities, exhibiting healthy behaviors, and gaining as much control over your life as possible. This chapter described a method you can use to learn to relax, which is one element of stress management.

# Part III

# HOW DO I PUT IT ALL TOGETHER?

> **What Is a Complete Physical Fitness Program?**
>
> **How Can I Increase Healthy and Decrease Unhealthy Actions?**
>
> **How Can I Prevent Injury Related to Exercise?**
>
> **How Can I Deal With Special Conditions?**

Part I helped you evaluate your current health status. Part II described the various components of fitness. This final part presents the contents of a complete physical fitness program as well as ways to modify your behavior, prevent injury, and deal with special personal and environmental conditions.

Chapter 11 defines the components of a fitness program. Chapter 12 takes you through recommended phases, starting with transition from sedentary living, going though months of conditioning, and leading to activities for people with high levels of fitness. If you follow these recommendations, you can increase your fitness level enjoyably and safely. Chapter 13 helps you figure out how many calories you are using in various activities. Chapter 14 deals with suggestions for helping you live a healthier life by adhering to your new exercise program and increasing healthful living in other areas of your life. Chapter 15 provides useful information on ways of exercising to reduce the chance of injury as well as what should be done to minimize injuries' effects when they do occur. Chapter 16 presents safe exercise practices for people with orthopedic or medical conditions that need special attention. Chapter 17 provides suggestions for exercising in varied environmental conditions. The final chapter looks at your exercise program from the broader perspective of a healthy life.

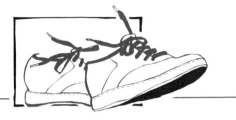

*Chapter*
## 11

# What Does a Complete Fitness Program Look Like?

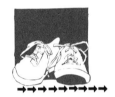

> **What Should I Consider in a Fitness Program?**
>
> **What Should I Include in a Workout?**

Part II gave you information on all the components of fitness summarized in Figure 11.1. This chapter begins with the two basic principles briefly introduced in chapter 7: *overload* and *specificity*.

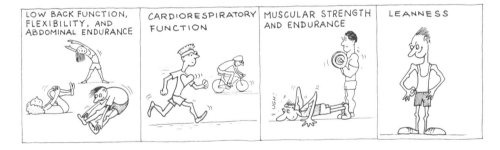

**Figure 11.1**  Fitness components.

## What Are the Principles of a Fitness Program?

Overload and specificity are related to improvement of all fitness components. In order for any body tissue to increase in function it must be exposed to a load greater than that to which it is accustomed; the tissue then gradually adapts to this load by increasing its size or function. The process of overload followed by adaptation is the basis of fitness and performance programs, and is called the *principle of overload*. Here is an example of this principle: A person whose heart function is weak due to years of sedentary living can overload the heart and entire cardiorespiratory system simply by slow walking.

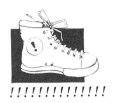

session is shortened due to lack of time, keep the warm-up and cool-down periods and reduce the time you spend in the main part of your workout.

- Warm-up, stretch, exercise, and cool-down.

### Why Should I Have Periodic Testing?

One of the major differences between fitness programs offered by health and fitness professionals and other "fitness" programs is the evaluation provided for you. A good fitness program provides periodic testing of the various fitness components. In this way you receive feedback about how you are doing as you move toward your goals. A general rule of thumb is to make about a 10% change over a 3-month period in the areas that need improvement. Once you achieve your goal, periodic testing provides evidence that you are holding your own. If you are doing your fitness program on your own, use the various self-tests for each fitness component that we have provided in Part II. You might want to test yourself at 3 months, 6 months, one year, and then annually to determine your progress.

### How Many Times Per Week Should I Work Out?

The recommended frequency of exercise to achieve both cardiovascular fitness as well as weight loss goals is three or four times per week—every other day. (The same recommendation holds for muscle strength and endurance programs.) Exercising fewer than three times a week requires a very high intensity of activity to achieve a cardiovascular training effect, and the higher intensity is associated with more injuries. In addition, it is difficult to achieve a weight loss goal when you exercise fewer than three times per week. If you exercise strenuously more than four times per week the risk of injury increases. The day-on, day-off routine seems to be optimal and makes an exercise program easy to schedule.

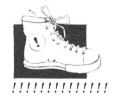

- Exercise three to four times a week on a day-on, day-off basis.

### How Much Total Work Should I Do During Each Workout?

Aim at expending 200 to 300 kcal per exercise session in order to achieve a cardiovascular training effect and meet body composition goals. The total caloric cost of a workout is determined by the duration and the intensity of the workout. Generally, you need about 30 to 40 minutes during a workout to achieve a 200 to 300 kcal expenditure when working at the appropriate intensity since some time is spent with flexibility and warm-up activities. If you do very light activity, then the duration has to be extended in order to achieve the 200 to 300 kcal goal.

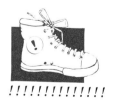

- Exercise long enough to expend about 200 to 300 kcal.

### How Do I Progress From Where I Am to Where I Should Be?

As we mentioned previously, it is important to *progress* from light, "too easy" exercise sessions to more intense exercise sessions. We feel that you should be able to walk 4 miles briskly before you undertake more strenuous activity. By achieving this goal you will have established a regular pattern of activity and made some body composition changes that will make the transition to more strenuous exercise easier. Figure 11.4 shows that the progression from walk to jog to run occurs over a period of months.

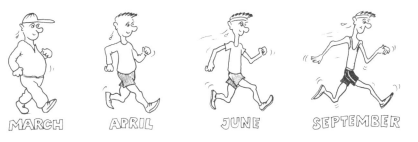

**Figure 11.4** Cardiorespiratory progression.

## How Hard Should I Work Out?

The intensity of exercise is best described by the overload it places on the cardiorespiratory system during a workout. The *threshold* needed to achieve the training effect is lower for the very sedentary (50% of maximal cardiorespiratory function) compared to the very fit (85% of maximal cardiorespiratory function). The primary way to judge exercise intensity is to see how high your heart rate is during the activity, since heart rate increases in a regular manner with exercise intensity. As a result of a variety of research studies you can estimate your appropriate exercise intensity by calculating a *target heart rate (THR) zone*. The THR zone represents the range of heart rate values that are *high enough to cause a training effect* yet *low enough to allow you to exercise long enough* to achieve the total work needed for a training effect.

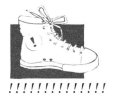

!!!!!!!!!!!!!!

The first step in calculating THR is to estimate your maximal heart rate. Complete the following:

---

**220 – age (years) = age-adjusted maximal heart rate**

**Example: For a 50-year-old person,**
  **220 – 50 = 170 beats per minute**

**Now use your own age:**
  **220 – _____ (years) = _____ beats per minute**

---

The second step is to calculate the THR zone:

---

**70% maximal heart rate = low end of THR zone**

**Example: 70% of 170 beats per minute = 119 beats per minute**

**For you, .70 × _____ beats per minute = _____ beats
  per minute**

**85% maximal heart rate = high end of THR zone**

**Example: 85% of 170 beats per minute = 145 beats per minute**

**For you: .85 × _____ beats per minute = _____ beats
  per minute**

---

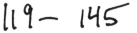

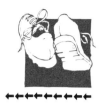

## Summary

Fitness changes are made by placing an overload on a tissue (muscle) or system (cardiovascular) and allowing an adaptation to occur over time. Fitness improvements are specific to the type of training; heavy resistance training leads to increases in muscle size and strength while light exercises done repeatedly result in endurance changes. A fitness program begins with an evaluation of health status and emphasizes the need to be regular and to start slowly. You should plan three or four workouts a week, at about 70 to 85% of maximal heart rate for 30 to 40 minutes per session to expend 200 to 300 kcal per session. Each session begins with a warm-up, concludes with a cool-down, and includes exercises to improve low back function and muscular endurance.

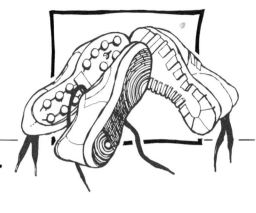

## Chapter
### *12*

# *What Activities Should I Include in My Fitness Program?*

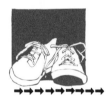

➜➜➜➜➜➜➜➜➜

| **What Are the Phases of a Fitness Program?** |
| **What Activities Can I Use in Each Phase?** |

In the previous chapter, we presented the general outline of a fitness program. In this chapter, we deal with more detailed steps for specific activities that lead to enhanced fitness, and we recommend that you progress through phases of your fitness program.

## Where Do I Start and How Do I Progress?

### Phase 1 — Regular Walking

As mentioned in the previous chapter, the first step in a fitness program is regular walking. This activity can range from very low to high intensity depending on the speed of the walk, and, as Figure 12.1 shows, it can be

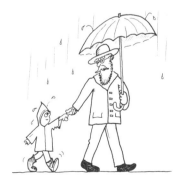

**Figure 12.1** Walking is for everyone.

done in any weather by anyone, young or old. We recommend that you achieve the ability to walk about 4 miles at a brisk pace without undue fatigue before moving on to more strenuous activities. A planned program to accomplish that will be presented shortly. If you can already do this level of activity without fatigue, go to Phase 2.

### Phase 2—Progress to Recommended Work Levels for Fitness Base

Once you have achieved the goal of the walking program, you may want to begin a walk/jog/run (or swim or bike) program to achieve higher levels of cardiorespiratory fitness. We emphasize the need to progress slowly from one stage of the program to the next in order to minimize muscle soreness and increase the probability of success. The THR zone will act as an intensity guide, helping you select your proper pace and the length of the first stages of the jog/walk intervals. Aim to be able to jog 3 miles in the THR zone. A typical walk/jog/run program follows our discussion of the program for walkers.

### Phase 3—Add Variety of Fitness Activities

After you have developed a fitness base that allows you to jog 3 miles comfortably, you are ready to undertake a variety of less controlled fitness games or activities. These often require some skill and have an inherently higher risk of injury. This phase is not for everyone and, of course, it is designed around your particular interests. We encourage you to develop new skills (an old dog can learn new tricks!), and become involved in a variety of activities. By doing so, you will have less risk of becoming sedentary. For example, if it is rainy and cold outside a jogger can substitute racquetball or participate in an aerobic dance class. A runner who hurts a knee can swim or cycle. Games provide a natural framework for establishing a socially supportive environment. Remember, you have to stay active to remain fit.

## What Are Some Different Activities Like?

In this section we will provide details of the walking, jogging, cycling, and exercise to music (often called "aerobics") programs, as well as comment on some other activities.

### What Should I Consider in Walking, Jogging, and Running Programs?

When you walk, one foot is always in contact with the ground. When you jog or run, there is a period of "flight" during which both feet are off the ground. The extra energy required to propel the body off the ground and to absorb the force of impact when landing makes jogging or running a better way to expend calories, but the probability of injury is higher as well. It is more difficult to distinguish jogging from running. A world class runner may "jog" through a warm-up at 7 miles per hour while a person of average fitness may be running all out at the same speed. Jogging usually refers to a submaximal running speed.

*Shoes.* Specialized walking shoes are now available from major shoe manufacturers catering to the growing market of walking enthusiasts. For most people, however, a comfortable pair of ordinary shoes offering reasonable side support is sufficient to start a walking program. Specialized walking shoes may be a reasonable investment for someone who has chosen walking as a primary activity. A good-quality pair of jogging/running shoes with the usual cushioning to absorb the shock of impact and the structural support to resist movement of the heels upon landing are also suitable for walking. So, if you are going to be moving from the walking to the jogging/running phases of a fitness program, an investment in a pair of good-quality running shoes is reasonable. We recommend that you buy your shoes at a store that specializes in athletic shoes and that you be fitted late in the day (when your feet are at their largest) wearing the same kind of socks you use during a workout.

*Clothing.*   Choose clothing that makes you feel as comfortable as possible during the exercise session. In hot weather wear loose-fitting, light-colored clothing and a hat with a brim if you are exercising in direct sunlight. Cotton fabrics are recommended—they allow sweat to evaporate. Be careful not to be taken in by advertising that suggests that by wearing plastic, nylon, or rubber clothing you will lose more weight when exercising in warm weather. The weight you lose is water weight, not fat weight, and wearing these fabrics can create a dangerous situation by making it more difficult to keep your body cool.

If you exercise outdoors in the cold weather, wear layers of clothing so that you can remove a layer or two as you warm up and begin to sweat. The idea is to not produce too much sweat, which can accelerate heat loss and result in hypothermia. Wool and polypropylene fabrics are recommended because they maintain their insulating qualities even when wet with sweat. A hat and mittens are recommended as you lose a great deal of heat from your head and hands. For those who tend to have cold hands, wearing a pair of polypropylene gloves inside mittens provides additional comfort. Emphasize comfort, not looks. Based on our observations of the outfits worn by some wintertime joggers, this approach to dressing for activity is certainly being followed!

*Location and Surface.*   The first consideration in choosing a workout site is *safety*. Walking is a good activity; walking in Central Park in New York City after dark is not healthful (nor smart!). Consider the traffic flow, lighting, and surface when you select an area. Low-traffic areas are more relaxing and reduce the chance of an accident. If you walk, jog, or run in the streets, be sure to run toward oncoming traffic so you can see what is ahead. In addition, wear bright clothing that is easily visible. Whether you believe you have the right of way or not, yield to traffic at every intersection or commercial driveway.

The surface should be relatively smooth, and you must be aware of cracks, holes, and debris to avoid sprains and strains. The hardness of the surface is not important for those who walk, as the force of impact is relatively low. For those who jog or run, the surface can influence the degree of comfort, especially if you have some arthritis in your ankles, knees, or hips. A soft surface like grass or a cushioned track will relieve some of the problems. When you jog on grass, however, be careful of roots and holes. Given the concern for injuries and safety, the area should be well lighted.

*Walking Program.*   The walking program shown in Table 12.1 on page 104 takes you from a very light level of activity to the point of being able to walk 60 minutes at a brisk pace. We have stated five rules at the top of the table. The most important rule is to not progress to the next stage until you are comfortable at the current stage. Don't be in a rush to get fit. Take your time and enjoy steady progress toward your goal. We recommend that you

## Table 12.1
## Walking Program

*Rules:*

1. Start at a level that is comfortable to you.
2. Be aware of new aches or pains.
3. Don't progress to next level if not comfortable.
4. Monitor heart rate and record it.
5. It would be healthful to walk at least every other day.

| Stage | Duration | Heart rate | Comments |
|-------|----------|------------|----------|
| 1 | 15 min | | |
| 2 | 20 min | | |
| 3 | 25 min | | |
| 4 | 30 min | | |
| 5 | 30 min | | |
| 6 | 30 min | | |
| 7 | 35 min | | |
| 8 | 40 min | | |
| 9 | 45 min | | |
| 10 | 45 min | | |
| 11 | 45 min | | |
| 12 | 50 min | | |
| 13 | 55 min | | |
| 14 | 60 min | | |
| 15 | 60 min | | |
| 16 | 60 min | | |
| 17 | 60 min | | |
| 18 | 60 min | | |
| 19 | 60 min | | |
| 20 | 60 min | | |

*Note.* From Howley and Franks (1986).

increase the *distance* you walk at a slow speed before you increase the *speed* that you walk. We have not stated a particular walking speed because what is comfortable for one person may be too fast for another. At the end of the walking program, when you can walk 4 miles or so at a brisk pace, you are ready to start the jogging program. However, as mentioned above, some of you will prefer to stay at the "brisk walk" stage of the walking program as your most intense activity. Walking with other(s) is enjoyable for many fitness participants. The main precaution when exercising together is to take care not to push each other to working beyond what is comfortable.

***Jogging Program.*** A jogging program is described in Table 12.2 (page 106). The first rule to follow is to complete the walking program. In addition, the first five levels of the program emphasize the need to mix walking with jogging to stay at the *low* end of the THR zone where you should perceive the exercise as being easy. This gradual transition will result in less muscle soreness. You might consider doing this program on a track, in a park, or on a very quiet street so that you will not have to be concerned with too much traffic or noise. In addition, you might find it more enjoyable if you jog with someone else. The time will fly by and you will have someone to help you along.

***Competition in Races.*** In almost every community there are opportunities to compete in running races—one-mile "fun runs" or social 10-kilometer (6.2 miles) runs. For people interested in jogging or running as a primary form of activity these runs can, and should, be fun. The focus of your attention in such runs should be on completing the course comfortably. As you become more fit you will be able to run the race in a shorter time. Remember, the focus of attention in this book is on becoming fit, not on achieving world-class status as a runner. Those who choose to emphasize competitive running, where the main goal is to run faster and faster, should expect more injuries and muscle soreness to accompany that endeavor. We advise a similar approach to walking races.

## What Would a Cycling Program Contain?

A cycling program can use a regular bicycle or one of the many stationary cycle ergometers found in fitness centers. Cycling is a good exercise alternative for people who do not like to jog or run and can also give relief to those who have joint tenderness. Adjust the seat height so that your knee has only a slight bend when your foot is at the bottom of a pedal swing. Table 12.3 (page 107) shows a cycling program that progresses in much the same way that the walk and jog programs did. The emphasis at the beginning of the program is on simply riding the equivalent of one or two miles three times per week. After that, work at the low end of the THR zone (around 70% of maximal heart rate) until you can comfortably do 15 to 25 minutes of activity. As you progress through the program, stay within your THR zone and do not advance to the next stage if you are not comfortable.

## How Can I Use Games and Sport for Fitness?

Games and some sports can be used in a fitness program, and for the reasons mentioned above, we encourage interested individuals to do so. However, we also recommend that a person first be able to move through the walking and the jogging programs. This is because those programs emphasize more controlled types of activity at an intensity that will help you achieve cardiovascular

**Table 12.2**

**Jogging Program**

*Rules:*

1. Complete the Walking Program before starting this program.

2. Begin each session with stretching and walking.

3. Be aware of new aches and pains.

4. Don't progress to next level if not comfortable.

5. Stay at low end of THR zone; record heart rate for each session.

6. Do program on a work-a-day, rest-a-day basis.

*Stage 1* Jog 10 steps, walk 10 steps. Repeat five times and take your heart rate. Stay within THR zone by increasing or decreasing walking phase. Do 20 to 30 min of activity.

*Stage 2* Jog 20 steps, walk 10 steps. Repeat five times and take your heart rate. Stay within THR zone by increasing or decreasing walking phase. Do 20 to 30 min of activity.

*Stage 3* Jog 30 steps, walk 10 steps. Repeat five times and take your heart rate. Stay within THR zone by increasing or decreasing walking phase. Do 20 to 30 min of activity.

*Stage 4* Jog 1 min, walk 10 steps. Repeat three times and take your heart rate. Stay within THR zone by increasing or decreasing walking phase. Do 20 to 30 min of activity.

*Stage 5* Jog 2 min, walk 10 steps. Repeat two times and take your heart rate. Stay within THR zone by increasing or decreasing walking phase. Do 30 min of activity.

*Stage 6* Jog 1 lap (400 m, or 440 yd) and check heart rate. Adjust pace during run to stay within the THR zone. If heart rate is still too high, go back to the Stage 5 schedule. Do 6 laps with a brief walk between each.

*Stage 7* Jog 2 laps and check heart rate. Adjust pace during run to stay within the THR zone. If heart rate is still too high, go back to Stage 6 activity. Do 6 laps with a brief walk between each.

*Stage 8* Jog 1 mi and check heart rate. Adjust pace during the run to stay within THR zone. Do 2 mi.

*Stage 9* Jog 2-3 mi continuously. Check heart rate at the end to ensure that you were within THR zone.

*Note.* From Howley and Franks (1986).

**Table 12.3**
## Cycling Program

*Rules:*

1. Start at a level that is comfortable for you.

2. Use either a regular bicycle or a stationary exercise cycle.

3. If you are starting at Stage 1, simply get used to riding 1 or 2 miles. Don't be concerned about time or reaching the lower end of your target heart rate (THR) zone.

| Stage | Distance (mi) | THR (% of max HR) | Time (min) | Frequency (days/week) |
|---|---|---|---|---|
| 1 | 1-2 | — | — | 3 |
| 2 | 1-2 | 60 | 8-12 | 3 |
| 3 | 3-5 | 60 | 15-25 | 3 |
| 4 | 6-8 | 70 | 25-35 | 3 |
| 5 | 6-8 | 70 | 25-35 | 4 |
| 6 | 10-15 | 70 | 40-60 | 4 |
| 7 | 10-15 | 80 | 35-50 | 4-5 |

*Note.* From Howley and Franks (1986).

fitness levels and change body composition to facilitate your involvement in a game. If you are not fit enough to play a game then the possibility of having fun is diminished and the possibility of injury is increased.

Games can help you achieve fitness if they are vigorous (i.e., you reach the THR zone) and are somewhat sustained so that you are exercising at the THR for 30 to 40 minutes. If you stand around or are excluded (e.g., sitting on the bench), games are not very useful in expending energy or raising morale. Many games require skill in order to participate in a meaningful way, and when one or both parties in a doubles game lack that skill, neither gets a workout. It is important that the participants have skill and are somewhat balanced in terms of ability to play. If you are interested in racquetball or tennis, realize that if a skill difference between the players exists, there is a good chance that you both will spend more time with flexibility exercises (picking up the ball) than with exercise that improves cardiorespiratory function. To make the transition from jogging to a particular game, you might continue your normal workouts and gradually learn the game.

Exercise leaders in some fitness programs use low-organized games as part of the fitness activities. These activities require minimal skill, and the fun level is maximal. The games can be controlled very easily to keep all participants in their respective THR zones, but you need to judge when the game is getting to be a little too much for you. The goal is to have fun and be fit; games certainly meet those requirements.

## What About Aquatic Activities?

You don't have to play games, run, or cycle to achieve a cardiorespiratory training effect. Swimming is an excellent alternative. Aquatic activities, however, include more than just swimming. You can walk, jog, or run across the pool; hold onto the side of the pool and do flexibility exercises; as well as play games in the water. Swimming or one of these other activities is a good choice if you have a chronic orthopedic problem or a recent injury that will not allow you to do your regular workout. Water supports your weight to relieve the load on ankles, knees, and hips while providing enough resistance to require the expenditure of a large number of calories and achieve THR.

*Target Heart Rate in Water.*   Your maximal heart rate is about 13 beats per minute *lower* when you are immersed in water. This shifts the THR zone back about 10 beats per minute since it is dependent on your maximal heart rate. So when you exercise in water you do not have to achieve the same THR value as you do on land to reach the proper exercise intensity that causes a training effect.

*Progression.*   Progress from low-intensity to higher-intensity activities in the pool in much the same way that you do on land. You can do flexibility activities by moving your legs forward, backward, and to the side in a gentle and easy motion while holding onto the side of the pool with one hand. You can also hang onto the side of the pool with both hands so that your body is floating and practice some of the kicking that is part of regular swimming. Those of you who cannot swim can walk or jog across the pool while doing a swimming stroke. Water offers enough resistance to this movement so that most people can achieve THR. Vary this by walking backward or skipping side to side while moving across the pool. You can use flotation devices to help yourself along while swimming; flotation offers a good deal of resistance while providing support. In this way even a nonswimmer can achieve a satisfying workout while "swimming" up and down the pool.

Swimming laps in the pool requires a certain level of skill—a poor swimmer will be exhausted at the end of one or two laps and will be unable to complete the duration of the workout needed to expend the necessary 200-300 kcal. You can learn to swim at any age and, besides the survival value of such a skill, swimming provides that special alternative when other exercise activities cannot be done due to injury, disease (like arthritis), or situation. Learn the simplest of strokes first, and gradually work up to others. Check THR during the swimming workout in much the same way as for running. The distance you have to swim to expend 300 or so kcal varies with the stroke used and the swimmer's skill level. A very rough rule of thumb is that a one-mile swim is equal to about 4 miles of jogging. Begin each workout with a gradual warm-up and finish with a cool-down. Table 12.4 (page 110) is a list of steps to follow in a swimming program.

You can start this swim program at any of the levels, depending on your skill and current fitness levels. Also, don't hesitate to vary the components to suit your needs. For example, you might like to jog four widths, swim four widths, and walk two widths, repeating the sequence to achieve 20 to 30 minutes of activity at the THR. Simply remember to take your time in making the transition to longer duration and more intense activities.

## What About Exercising to Music?

One of the best things to happen to fitness exercises in the past 20 years was setting them to music. It has provided an exercise opportunity for people who do not like to jog or run. In addition, exercising to music provides one less excuse to those of us who would skip our exercise sessions because it is (pick one) too hot, too cold, raining, and so on.

*Advantages.* Music provides a sense of pace and the motivation to keep at it, in contrast to other, more isolated activities such as cycling, jogging on a treadmill, or swimming laps in a pool. The pace can be varied by the tempo of the music, which becomes a distraction from the exercise as you listen to the changing rhythms. In addition, musical exercise sessions offer a better balance of activities to achieve fitness goals in flexibility, muscular endurance, and cardiorespiratory endurance. Generally speaking, you will have no problem reaching your THR during a session. In fact, you may find it easy to reach your THR, and we recommend that you make sure you do too little rather than too much as you begin this type of exercise. Put the emphasis on enjoying the session, not competing with others, either in the types of steps you use or in continuing when your body is telling you to slow down. As we mentioned earlier, the idea of "no pain, no gain," still heard in some health clubs, is wrong! "Train, don't strain" is more appropriate and will bring you more benefits in the long run.

*Disadvantages.* The reason for doing too little rather than too much is that exercise-to-music programs lead to their share of injuries. The routines tend to isolate smaller muscle groups and skeletal structures. In addition, people may start this kind of activity program before they are ready. We recommend that you achieve a minimum level of fitness (equivalent to jogging 3 miles at THR) before undertaking this kind of activity. Further, we suggest that you vary this kind of exercise with others that do not put as much stress on joints, like cycling and swimming.

*Level.* Fitness centers now offer a wider variety of exercise-to-music classes than they did in the past. This is partly in response to the incidence of injuries

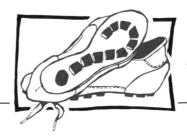

## Chapter
## 13

# How Many Calories Am I Using?

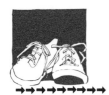

**How Can I Determine How Much Energy I Am Using?**
**What Are the Caloric Costs of Different Activities?**

We have discussed how important modifications in both diet and exercise are in achieving weight loss goals and maintaining the new weight. It is often recommended that you burn 200 to 300 kcal during each exercise session. Though most of you are familiar with the caloric costs of food, as values are usually printed on food packages, such is not the case for the caloric costs of physical activity. Since this is quite an important bit of information, it should be no surprise that researchers have developed various methods to measure the energy costs of physical activity.

## What Are Ways to Measure Energy Use?

When we use oxygen, energy is produced to contract a muscle, initiate a nerve impulse, repair a bone, or carry out any number of cellular functions. Oxygen goes from the lungs to the blood and finally to the tissues where it is used. For each liter of oxygen used, the body produces about 5 kcal. Knowing this, it is possible to measure the amount of energy produced during the course of a day simply by measuring oxygen consumption. On the basis of these measurements we are able to estimate the amount of energy a person uses for different activities and provide an overall estimate of what a person might expend in one day. When we are sitting at rest we produce about one kcal per hour for every kilogram (2.2 pounds) of body weight. The value of one kcal per kilogram per hour is one resting metabolic unit or *1 MET*. METs have already been used to quantify your CRF in chapter 6. METs are also used in expressing the energy costs of activities; for example, running at 6 miles per hour requires 10 METs, or 10 times the rate of energy expended at rest. Before discussing the energy costs of physical activity, however, we need to focus on the energy associated with sitting at rest, the largest energy-producing task in the lives of most people! Given that we produce about one kcal of energy per kilogram of body weight per hour at rest, you can estimate your resting energy expenditure (also called basal metabolic rate, or BMR) by doing the following:

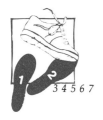

---

**1. Multiply 24 kcal times body weight in kilograms (pounds ÷ 2.2)**

or

**2. Multiply 11 kcal times body weight in pounds**

---

For example, for a 150-pound person, 150 pounds × 11 kcal per pound = 1,650 kcal. This, of course, represents only resting energy expenditure. To obtain an estimate of overall energy expenditure, you must add the energy cost of other activities that you do. This is done by adding from 400 to 800 kcal, depending on whether you are sedentary or very active. So, if our 150-pound person is sedentary, the estimated total energy expenditure is 2,050 kcal per day (1,650 kcal + 400 kcal). Remember that this is a rough estimate and like any estimate may be too high or too low for you. Use it as a guide, but if you find yourself gaining weight even though you are eating just enough food to meet your estimated energy expenditure, decrease your estimate about 10% and see if you can maintain weight on that new estimate. Keep in mind that if you reduce your caloric intake to a very low level your body responds by decreasing its resting metabolic rate to protect its limited energy stores. In such a circumstance the above formula will result in an overestimation of energy expenditure.

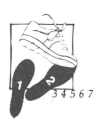

---

**Estimate Your Daily Energy Expenditure**

1. **Determine resting metabolic rate:**

   **Multiply 11 by your body weight:**
   11 × _____ pounds = _____ kcal

2. **Select 400 kcal if sedentary, 600 kcal if moderately active, and 800 kcal if active**

3. **Daily energy expenditure:**
   Total from (line 1) _____ kcal + Selection from
   (line 2) _____ kcal = _____ kcal

---

## What Are the Energy Costs of Common Activities?

The techniques used to measure energy expenditure at rest have also been used to measure the energy required to do certain activities. This section presents information on the energy required for some of the most common activities associated with physical fitness programs.

### Walking

We recommend a walking program for anyone who has not been active for some time. The program provides stages of gradually increasing duration and intensity and is the lead-in to a jogging/running program. For many people, the walking program may be all they wish or need to do to maintain fitness. Walking has the advantage that it can be done anywhere, any time, by virtually anyone. Given this, it is no surprise that we know a great deal about the energy cost of walking. Scientists have studied the energy cost of walking indoors using a treadmill, and outdoors on a track, beach, or farm. Walking on a beach or across a plowed field requires more energy than walking at the same speed on a flat, firm surface. Because most people exercise on a firm surface, however, we will discuss the energy costs of walking with reference to this situation.

Table 13.1 shows the energy required to walk at different speeds. The values are given in METs, or multiples of the resting metabolic rate. Not surprisingly, the energy cost of walking increases with the speed of walking; however, the rate of increase is higher at the higher speeds. For example, when walking speed increases from 2 to 3 miles per hour the energy required increases from 2.5 to 3.3 METs. But going from 4 to 5 miles per hour requires an increase from 4.9 to 7.9 METs. Also, the energy cost of walking (or jogging or running, as we'll see later) increases with the weight of the individual. As you can see in Table 13.1, the 110-pound person expends fewer calories per minute compared with the 140-pound person at any given speed. As we mentioned earlier, walking can be done by just about anyone to have a fitness effect. The very sedentary individual can walk at slow speeds and achieve THR while the relatively fit individual can walk at high speeds where the elevated energy requirement allows THR to be reached.

**Table 13.1**
**Energy Costs of Walking (kcal/Minute)**

| Body weight (lb) | Miles per hour/METs | | | | | | |
|---|---|---|---|---|---|---|---|
| | 2.0/2.5 | 2.5/2.9 | 3.0/3.3 | 3.5/3.7 | 4.0/4.9 | 4.5/6.2 | 5.0/7.9 |
| 110 | 2.1 | 2.4 | 2.8 | 3.1 | 4.1 | 5.2 | 6.6 |
| 120 | 2.3 | 2.6 | 3.0 | 3.4 | 4.4 | 5.6 | 7.2 |
| 130 | 2.5 | 2.9 | 3.2 | 3.6 | 4.8 | 6.1 | 7.8 |
| 140 | 2.7 | 3.1 | 3.5 | 3.9 | 5.2 | 6.6 | 8.4 |
| 150 | 2.8 | 3.3 | 3.7 | 4.2 | 5.6 | 7.0 | 9.0 |
| 160 | 3.0 | 3.5 | 4.0 | 4.5 | 5.9 | 7.5 | 9.6 |
| 170 | 3.2 | 3.7 | 4.2 | 4.8 | 6.3 | 8.0 | 10.2 |
| 180 | 3.4 | 4.0 | 4.5 | 5.0 | 6.7 | 8.4 | 10.8 |
| 190 | 3.6 | 4.2 | 4.7 | 5.3 | 7.0 | 8.9 | 11.4 |
| 200 | 3.8 | 4.4 | 5.0 | 5.6 | 7.4 | 9.4 | 12.0 |
| 210 | 4.0 | 4.6 | 5.2 | 5.9 | 7.8 | 9.9 | 12.6 |
| 220 | 4.2 | 4.8 | 5.5 | 6.2 | 8.2 | 10.3 | 13.2 |

## Jogging and Running

Many people jog and run to achieve their fitness and weight loss goals. The energy requirement of jogging is about *twice* that of walking at 3 miles per hour, but is nearly the same as walking at 5 miles per hour. Table 13.2 on page 116 shows the energy required to jog or run at different speeds. As you can see, the energy requirement increases with increasing speed, but the increase in the energy cost from one speed to the next is similar at slow and fast speeds, about 1.5 METs per mile-per-hour increase in speed. This proportional increase in energy cost means that when you jog a mile at 6 miles an hour (10 minutes per mile) you will finish the mile twice as fast as when jogging at 3 miles per hour, but the energy required per mile is about the same. This is a bothersome point for many people, but it is true. If one person works at 10 METs (about a 6 mile-per-hour jog) for 20 minutes, and another works at 5 METs (about a 3 mile-per-hour jog) for 40 minutes, they both expend about the same amount of energy. We will discuss this topic further in the next section.

**Table 13.2**
**Energy Costs of Jogging and Running (kcal/Minute)**

| Body weight (lb) | Miles per hour/METs | | | | | | | |
|---|---|---|---|---|---|---|---|---|
| | 3.0/5.6 | 4.0/7.1 | 5.0/8.7 | 6.0/10.2 | 7.0/11.7 | 8.0/13.3 | 9.0/14.8 | 10.0/16.3 |
| 110 | 4.7 | 5.9 | 7.2 | 8.5 | 9.8 | 11.1 | 12.3 | 13.6 |
| 120 | 5.1 | 6.4 | 7.9 | 9.3 | 10.6 | 12.1 | 13.4 | 14.8 |
| 130 | 5.5 | 7.0 | 8.6 | 10.0 | 11.5 | 13.1 | 14.6 | 16.1 |
| 140 | 5.9 | 7.5 | 9.2 | 10.8 | 12.4 | 14.1 | 15.7 | 17.3 |
| 150 | 6.4 | 8.1 | 9.9 | 11.6 | 13.3 | 15.1 | 16.8 | 18.5 |
| 160 | 6.8 | 8.6 | 10.5 | 12.4 | 14.2 | 16.1 | 17.9 | 19.8 |
| 170 | 7.2 | 9.1 | 11.2 | 13.1 | 15.1 | 17.1 | 19.1 | 21.0 |
| 180 | 7.6 | 9.7 | 11.8 | 13.9 | 15.9 | 18.1 | 20.2 | 22.2 |
| 190 | 8.1 | 10.2 | 12.5 | 14.7 | 16.8 | 19.1 | 21.3 | 23.5 |
| 200 | 8.5 | 10.8 | 13.2 | 15.4 | 17.7 | 20.1 | 22.4 | 24.7 |
| 210 | 8.9 | 11.3 | 13.8 | 16.2 | 18.6 | 21.1 | 23.5 | 25.9 |
| 220 | 9.3 | 11.8 | 14.5 | 17.0 | 19.5 | 22.2 | 24.7 | 27.2 |

## Caloric Costs of Walking Versus Running One Mile

In spite of the vast amount of information available regarding the energy costs of walking and running, a good deal of misunderstanding exists. We still hear claims that the energy cost of walking one mile is equal to that of running the same distance. Although this is generally not the case, walking can be just about as good as running for expending calories. We will try to explain this apparent contradiction.

Table 13.3 shows the energy cost of walking one mile, and Table 13.4 shows the energy cost of running one mile. Given that energy cost is dependent on body weight (heavier people require more energy to travel one mile than lighter people do), the caloric cost is given for different body weights. The table contains two numbers for each weight, one expressing the *gross* cost of the activity and the other expressing the *net* cost. Gross cost includes the resting metabolic rate (the cost of just sitting around), while net cost subtracts this quantity out. For weight control programs it is important to use the net cost of an activity as it measures the energy used over and above that of sitting around. When moving at slow to moderate speeds (2 to 3.5 miles per hour), the net cost of walking a mile is about half that of jogging or running a mile. This means that the person who jogs a mile at 3 miles per hour will be working at twice the metabolic rate of someone who walks at the same speed and, of course, the heart rate response will be higher as well. Because most people who walk move at these slower speeds, it is important to remember that the energy cost per mile is half that of running.

**Table 13.3**
**Gross and Net (Gross/Net) Cost in kcal/Mile for Walking**

| Body weight (lb) | Miles per hour | | | | | | |
|---|---|---|---|---|---|---|---|
| | 2.0 | 2.5 | 3.0 | 3.5 | 4.0 | 4.5 | 5.0 |
| 110 | 64/39 | 58/39 | 54/39 | 53/39 | 60/48 | 68/57 | 79/69 |
| 120 | 69/42 | 63/42 | 59/42 | 57/42 | 66/52 | 75/63 | 86/75 |
| 130 | 75/45 | 68/45 | 64/45 | 62/45 | 71/57 | 81/68 | 93/81 |
| 140 | 80/49 | 73/49 | 69/49 | 67/49 | 77/61 | 87/73 | 100/88 |
| 150 | 87/52 | 79/52 | 74/52 | 72/52 | 82/65 | 93/78 | 108/94 |
| 160 | 92/56 | 84/56 | 79/56 | 76/56 | 88/70 | 100/84 | 115/100 |
| 170 | 98/59 | 90/59 | 84/59 | 81/59 | 93/74 | 106/89 | 122/107 |
| 180 | 104/63 | 95/63 | 89/63 | 86/63 | 99/78 | 112/94 | 129/113 |
| 190 | 110/66 | 100/66 | 94/66 | 91/66 | 104/83 | 118/99 | 136/119 |
| 200 | 115/70 | 105/70 | 99/70 | 95/70 | 110/87 | 124/104 | 144/125 |
| 210 | 121/73 | 111/73 | 104/73 | 100/73 | 115/92 | 131/110 | 151/132 |
| 220 | 127/77 | 116/77 | 109/77 | 105/77 | 121/96 | 137/115 | 158/138 |

**Table 13.4**
**Gross and Net (Gross/Net) Cost in kcal/Mile for Jogging and Running**

| Body weight (lb) | Miles per hour | | | | | | |
|---|---|---|---|---|---|---|---|
| | 3.0 | 4.0 | 5.0 | 6.0 | 7.0 | 8.0 | 9.0 | 10.0 |
| 110 | 93/77 | 89/77 | 86/77 | 84/77 | 84/77 | 83/77 | 82/77 | 81/77 |
| 120 | 101/83 | 97/83 | 94/83 | 92/83 | 92/83 | 90/83 | 89/83 | 89/83 |
| 130 | 110/90 | 105/90 | 102/90 | 100/90 | 99/90 | 98/90 | 97/90 | 96/90 |
| 140 | 118/97 | 113/97 | 110/97 | 108/97 | 107/97 | 106/97 | 104/97 | 104/97 |
| 150 | 127/104 | 121/104 | 118/104 | 115/104 | 114/104 | 113/104 | 112/104 | 111/104 |
| 160 | 135/111 | 129/111 | 125/111 | 123/111 | 122/111 | 121/111 | 119/111 | 119/111 |
| 170 | 144/118 | 137/118 | 133/118 | 131/118 | 130/118 | 128/118 | 127/118 | 126/118 |
| 180 | 152/125 | 146/125 | 141/125 | 146/132 | 145/132 | 143/132 | 141/132 | 141/132 |
| 190 | 161/132 | 154/132 | 149/132 | 146/132 | 145/132 | 143/132 | 141/132 | 141/132 |
| 200 | 169/139 | 162/139 | 157/139 | 154/139 | 153/139 | 151/139 | 149/139 | 148/139 |
| 210 | 177/146 | 170/146 | 165/146 | 161/146 | 160/146 | 158/146 | 156/146 | 155/146 |
| 220 | 186/153 | 178/153 | 173/153 | 169/153 | 168/153 | 166/153 | 164/153 | 163/153 |

However, if we now look at very high walking speeds of 5 miles per hour (one mile in 12 minutes) we see that the net energy cost of walking is similar to that of jogging or running. If you try it you will find that your heart rate response may actually be higher than it would be if you were running at that speed. If you can walk at these high speeds you can easily reach your THR and expend kcal at about the same rate as during running.

You may now wonder why we stated that walking can be just about as good as jogging in expending calories. When a person jogs or runs, it takes time to leave the office or home, change clothes, gradually warm up, shower afterward, change clothes again, and return to the office or home. Of the 60 minutes that may be dedicated to a workout only about 30 minutes may actually be spent running; the remainder is spent somewhat near the resting level. A person who walks for exercise can simply get up, perhaps change shirts, and get moving. Almost the entire 60 minutes is spent in activity. What

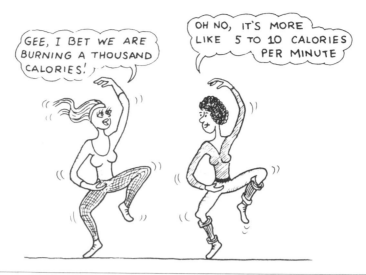

**Figure 13.2** Energy cost of exercise to music.

## Rope Skipping

Rope skipping can be done indoors or out, requires little formal equipment, and can be an effective *part* of a fitness program for people with high levels of fitness and regular activity. We emphasize the latter point because rope skipping places a load primarily on the lower leg, involves smaller muscle groups than walking and running, and causes a disproportionately higher heart rate response. Overdoing this activity, especially if you are at the beginning of a fitness program, is inappropriate. Our concern is based on the energy cost of rope skipping (Table 13.6), where we see that even a very slow skipping rate (60 to 80 turns per minute), requires 9 METs and a heart rate of more than 150 beats per minute in young fit subjects. Skipping at 120 turns per minute increases the energy cost to only 11 METs. As a result, skipping is not a "graded" activity—even the lowest skipping rate (60 to 80 turns per minute) requires an energy expenditure equal to or higher than the cardiorespiratory fitness of many sedentary people.

**Table 13.6**
**Gross Energy Cost of Rope Skipping (kcal/Minute)**

| Body weight (lb) | Slow skipping | Fast skipping |
| --- | --- | --- |
| 110 | 7.5 | 9.2 |
| 120 | 8.2 | 10.0 |
| 130 | 8.9 | 10.9 |
| 140 | 9.5 | 11.7 |
| 150 | 10.2 | 12.5 |
| 160 | 10.9 | 13.4 |
| 170 | 11.6 | 14.2 |
| 180 | 12.3 | 15.0 |
| 190 | 13.0 | 15.9 |
| 200 | 13.6 | 16.7 |
| 210 | 14.3 | 17.5 |
| 220 | 15.0 | 18.4 |

### Swimming

Swimming is an excellent activity because it involves the large muscle groups and provides little trauma to joints while expending a relatively large number of calories. However, predicting the caloric cost of swimming is difficult because caloric cost is dependent on the type of stroke used, swimming speed, and the skill of the swimmer. A poor swimmer must expend greater quantities of energy just to stay afloat or move at a slow pace, while a highly skilled swimmer expends very few calories doing the same thing. As a rule of thumb, *the net caloric cost of swimming one mile has been estimated to be about four times that of running one mile* (400 kcal vs. 100 kcal). Table 13.7 shows the estimated caloric cost per mile of swimming the front crawl for men and women. Because of their greater buoyancy associated with higher body fatness, women expend fewer calories per mile than men, independent of skill level. It should be noted that the maximal heart rate is about 13 beats per minute lower in water than on land. For this reason reduce your THR about 10 beats per minute from that calculated by the 220 − age formula.

**Table 13.7**
**Caloric Cost Per Mile (kcal/Mile) of Swimming the Front Crawl**
**for Men and Women by Skill Level**

| Skill level | Women | Men |
|---|---|---|
| Competitive | 180 | 280 |
| Skilled | 260 | 360 |
| Average | 300 | 440 |
| Unskilled | 360 | 560 |
| Poor | 440 | 720 |

*Note.* Adapted from Holmer (1980).

### Summary of the Energy Costs of Activities

We have presented only a few of the most common activities used in fitness programs. Table 13.8 (pages 122-123) provides some details about other activities in which you may be involved. The MET level gives some indication of the relative intensity of each activity and should provide some guidance as to whether you should include it in your activity program. Remember, to select activities that will keep you in the THR zone and will expend calories. Caloric expenditures are listed for three body weights, indicating an approximate range of energy expenditures associated with each activity.

# Is There An Easy Way to Estimate Energy Expenditure?

Estimating energy expenditure can be simplified in such a way that you can obtain a reasonable figure without having to consult all sorts of tables and figures. The estimate is based on the observation that when you are working in your THR zone you are at about 70% of your cardiorespiratory fitness value. For example, if you have a CRF value of 10 METs you would be exercising at about 7 METs while in the THR zone. Because 1 MET is equal

## Table 13.8
## Summary of Measured Energy Cost of Various Physical Activities

| Activity | METs | kcal/[kg × min] | kcal/hour 50 kg (110 lb) | 70 kg (154 lb) | 90 kg (198 lb) |
|---|---|---|---|---|---|
| Archery | 3-4 | .050-.066 | 150-200 | 210-280 | 270-360 |
| Backpacking | 5-11 | .083-.183 | 250-550 | 350-770 | 450-990 |
| Badminton | 4-9 | .066-.150 | 200-450 | 280-630 | 380-810 |
| Basketball | 3-12 | .050-.200 | 150-600 | 210-840 | 270-1080 |
| Billiards | 2.5 | .042 | 125 | 175 | 225 |
| Bowling | 2-4 | .033-.066 | 100-200 | 140-280 | 180-360 |
| Boxing | 8-13 | .133-.216 | 400-650 | 560-910 | 720-1170 |
| Canoeing, rowing, and kayaking | 3-8 | .050-.133 | 150-400 | 210-560 | 270-720 |
| Cricket | 4-7 | .066-.177 | 200-350 | 280-490 | 360-630 |
| Croquet | 3.5 | .058 | 175 | 245 | 315 |
| Cycling | 3-8 + | .050-.133 + | 150-400 + | 210-560 + | 270-720 + |
| Dancing | | | | | |
|   Social/tap | 3-7 | .050-.117 | 150-350 | 210-490 | 270-630 |
|   Aerobic (see p. 119) | 4-10 | .066-.167 | 200-500 | 280-700 | 360-900 |
| Fencing | 6-10 | .100-.167 | 300-500 | 420-700 | 540-900 |
| Field hockey | 8 | .133 | 400 | 560 | 720 |
| Fishing | | | | | |
|   From bank | 2-4 | .033-.066 | 100-200 | 140-280 | 180-360 |
|   Wading | 5-6 | .083-.100 | 250-300 | 350-420 | 450-540 |
| Football (touch) | 6-10 | .100-.167 | 300-500 | 420-700 | 540-900 |
| Golf | | | | | |
|   Power cart | 2-3 | .033-.050 | 100-150 | 140-210 | 180-270 |
|   Pull/carry clubs | 4-7 | .066-.117 | 200-350 | 280-490 | 360-630 |
| Handball | 8-12 | .133-.200 | 400-600 | 560-840 | 720-1080 |
| Hiking | 3-7 | .050-.117 | 150-350 | 210-490 | 270-670 |
| Horseback riding | 3-8 | .050-.133 | 150-400 | 210-560 | 270-720 |
| Horseshoe pitching | 2-3 | .033-.050 | 100-150 | 140-210 | 180-270 |
| Hunting small game (bow/gun) | 3-7 | .050-.117 | 150-350 | 210-490 | 270-630 |
| Jogging (see pp. 115-117) | | | | | |
| Mountain climbing | 5-10 | .083-.167 | 250-500 | 350-700 | 450-900 |
| Paddleball/racquetball | 8-12 | .133-.200 | 400-600 | 560-840 | 720-1080 |
| Rope jumping (see p. 120) | 9-12 | .15 -.20 | 450-600 | 630-840 | 810-1080 |
| Running (see p. 117) | | | | | |
| Sailing | 2-5 | .033-.083 | 100-250 | 140-350 | 180-450 |
| Scuba diving | 5-10 | .083-.167 | 250-500 | 350-700 | 450-900 |
| Shuffleboard | 2-3 | .033-.050 | 100-150 | 140-210 | 180-270 |
| Skating (ice and roller) | 5-8 | .083-.133 | 250-400 | 350-560 | 450-720 |
| Skiing (snow) | | | | | |
|   Downhill | 5-8 | .083-.133 | 250-400 | 350-560 | 450-720 |
|   Cross-country | 6-12 | .100-.200 | 300-600 | 420-840 | 540-1080 |
| Skiing (water) | 5-7 | .083-.117 | 250-350 | 350-490 | 450-630 |
| Sledding, tobogganing | 4-8 | .066-.113 | 200-400 | 280-560 | 360-720 |
| Snowshoeing | 7-14 | .117-.233 | 350-700 | 490-980 | 630-1260 |

| Activity | METs | kcal/[kg × min] | kcal/hour | | |
|---|---|---|---|---|---|
| | | | 50 kg (110 lb) | 70 kg (154 lb) | 90 kg (198 lb) |
| Squash | 8-12 | .133-.200 | 400-600 | 560-840 | 720-1080 |
| Soccer | 5-12 | .083-.200 | 250-600 | 350-840 | 450-1080 |
| Swimming (see p. 121) | | | | | |
| Table tennis | 3-5 | .050-.083 | 150-250 | 210-350 | 270-450 |
| Tennis | 4-9 | .066-.150 | 200-450 | 280-630 | 360-810 |
| Volleyball (recreational) | 3-6 | .050-.100 | 150-300 | 210-420 | 270-540 |
| Walking (see pp. 114-117) | | | | | |

*Note.* Adapted from the American College of Sports Medicine (1980) and McArdle, Katch, and Katch (1981).

to 1 kcal per kilogram per hour, a person working at 7 METs is working at 7 kcal per kilogram per hour. If that person weighs 70 kilograms (154 pounds) it means that 490 kcal are expended per hour in the activity. If the activity lasts only 30 minutes, then half that, or 245 kcal, are expended. Therefore, by knowing your maximal MET value (CRF value) you can obtain a reasonable estimate of how many kcal you are expending. Table 13.9 is based on those calculations for a 30-minute workout. Locate your estimated CRF on the left and look across the table to your approximate body weight to find your estimated energy expenditure for a 30 minute workout at your THR.

**Table 13.9**
**Estimated Energy Expenditure (kcal) for 30 Minutes of Exercise
at 70% Cardiorespiratory Fitness Value (CRF)[a]
for Persons of Different Body Weights**

| 70% CRF (METs) | Body weight [kg (lb)] | | |
|---|---|---|---|
| | 50 (110) | 70 (154) | 90 (198) |
| 14.0 | 350 | 490 | 630 |
| 12.6 | 315 | 441 | 567 |
| 11.2 | 280 | 392 | 504 |
| 9.8 | 245 | 343 | 441 |
| 8.4 | 210 | 294 | 378 |
| 7.0 | 175 | 245 | 315 |
| 5.6 | 140 | 196 | 252 |
| 4.2 | 105 | 147 | 189 |

*Note.* Adapted from Sharkey (1984).

[a]See chapter 6 for an explanation of the term.

## Summary

This chapter described the caloric costs of a variety of activities. You can determine your daily energy expenditure by multiplying your body weight by 11 and adding from 400 to 800 kcal based on your activity level. At normal speeds, it costs about twice as much energy to run as to walk a set distance.

Exercise to music can use as much energy as walking or running depending on how intensely you exercise. To expend the same amount of energy as it takes to run a set distance, you have to cycle about four times or swim about one fourth that distance.

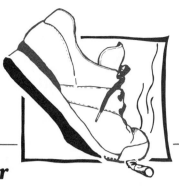

## Chapter
## *14*

# *How Can I Modify My Behaviors?*

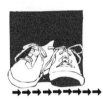

> **How Can I Change Things I Don't Like About Myself?**
>
> **How Can I Increase Exercise?**
>
> **How Can I Stay With My Exercise Program?**
>
> **How Can I Stop Smoking?**
>
> **How Can I Reduce Drinking?**
>
> **How Can I Change to a Healthier Diet?**
>
> **How Can I Cope With Stress?**

Do you exercise at least three times per week at a moderate intensity for 30 to 40 minutes each workout? Do you smoke? Do you have more than a couple of drinks per week? Do you take other drugs or medicine on a regular basis? Is your weight what it should be? Do you eat a well-balanced diet? Are you able to cope with day-to-day stressors? Can you deal with big emotional problems when they arise? Do you rely on eating, drinking, and/or drugs when problems arise? If your answers to these questions reflect a healthy life-style, then you can skip this chapter. Most of us, however, have one or more habits that prevent our achieving our highest possible levels of fitness and health. In fact, as a society we could make great strides in public health if we changed several aspects of the typical U.S.A. lifestyle.

If you have thought about changing the way you live so you can be healthier, then this chapter can help you. The chapter focuses on five behaviors that are directly related to positive health. For many people, the healthy life includes one or more of the following: reduction of smoking, alcohol intake, weight, and stress; and increasing exercise. The first part of the chapter includes general points to consider in trying to modify any behavior. The rest of the chapter discusses the reasons for specific unhealthy behaviors and ways to help you deal with them.

125

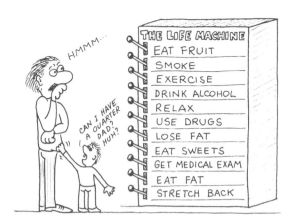

**Figure 14.1** The choice is yours.

## How Can I Change My Behavior?

Later in the chapter, we discuss the problems of inactivity, smoking, alcoholism, excess fat, and stress and recommend some specific procedures for resolving them. In addition we include some general steps that can help you adopt healthy behaviors. This general plan has several components, but you won't necessarily use each step for every habit you want to change. A procedure that helps you to resolve one particular problem may not work for someone else, and it may not help you resolve other problems. The steps outlined in Table 14.1 provide a general plan of steps that can be eliminated, added to, or modified depending on what works for you. The general plan is also a preview of the procedures to modify specific behaviors that we discuss in later portions of this chapter.

As you begin to make changes in your life, don't feel that you have to do it alone—ask for help. Choose someone who is a good role model for the desired behavior and who will be supportive of you as you make changes.

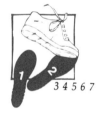

**Table 14.1**
**General Model for Changing Behavior**

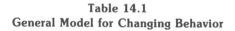

| Step | Activity |
|------|----------|
| 1 | Acknowledge desire to change |
| 2 | Analyze history of problem |
| 3 | Record current behavior |
| 4 | Analyze current status |
| 5 | Set long-term goals |
| 6 | Set short-term goals |
| 7 | Sign contract with friend(s) |
| 8 | List many possible strategies that could be used |
| 9 | Select one or two strategies to use |
| 10 | Learn new coping skills |
| 11 | Establish regular contact with helper |
| 12 | Once goal reached, outline potential maintenance problems |
| 13 | Learn new coping skills |
| 14 | Maintain periodic contact with helper |

*Note.* Adapted from Howley and Franks (1986).

Your fitness instructor, a counselor, or a close friend are good choices to enlist to help you throughout the process. The first step is to analyze the problem. Analysis includes facing such questions as when the behavior started, what the conditions were, why it continues, when it last happened, and under what conditions. Both you and your helper need to reach a mutual understanding of the problem. Collecting some baseline data concerning the extent of the behavior over a period of several days often aids this analysis. After the initial analysis, you should be able to clearly describe the current status of the problem.

Once you have analyzed the past and present, address the future by discussing your goals. Goal statements concern future conditions and often include time constraints. You suggest your desired goal, and the helper assists in making the goal realistic and clear. If you desire a large amount of behavior change, subgoals are advisable. Achieving the goal of successful behavior for a single day may lead to two successful days, then three, a week, and so on. To increase the chances of achieving the goal, a reward can be given contingent on the successful accomplishment of the goal. You receive the reward only if you reach the goal.

Another procedure that has helped individuals achieve goals is signing a contract. A written agreement, specifying the conditions to be met and the rewards or consequences if it is or is not met, is more successful if it is made between the individual who wants to change and a close friend. Some contracts are for taking positive steps *to do something* (e.g., beginning exercise—see Table 14.2). Other contracts are to avoid negative behavior and *to quit doing something* (e.g., stopping smoking—see Table 14.3). In some cases, contracts are made among a group of individuals who can provide support to each other and increase everyone's level of commitment.

Once you have analyzed a problem and agreed to a goal, the next step is to determine a plan for reaching the goal. The first step in developing a plan is for you and your helper to brainstorm—list as many different plans as possible without taking time to evaluate each one. From this list, pick the one or two strategies that seem to have the best chance of success. Depending on the strategy you select, you may need to learn new coping behaviors, such as new social skills, increased professional competence, and how to relax or be assertive. The particular coping behaviors you focus upon depend upon what goals and strategies you select.

If you have had difficulty in changing a certain behavior in the past, you may feel fearful and helpless about trying to change again. Express these feelings to your helper and ask for help in going forward in spite of these feelings. After you have reached an initial goal, a very difficult stage is entered: namely, how can you maintain long-term results? You need to recognize the environmental conditions under which old behaviors are likely to occur. Being able to recognize the onset of these potentially dangerous conditions increases the likelihood that you can take steps to avoid them. Long-term contact between you and your helper can maintain the change over time. This contact can become less frequent as your new behavior(s) becomes part of your lifestyle.

## How Can I Increase and Maintain Exercise?

There is general agreement that exercise is good for people. The 1990 health objectives for the U.S. include a threefold increase in appropriate aerobic exercise in the adult population. Exercise seems to be good both physiologically and psychologically. Chapters 11 and 12 dealt with specific factors (e.g., intensity) needed for improvement in health-related fitness as well as a variety of activities that can be used for fitness.

The current emphasis on and interest in fitness has brought many people (like you) into fitness programs. A major problem for you will be sticking with it, as in many programs up to 50% of participants quit within 6 months. People more likely to drop out include those who smoke, have low self-motivation, lack social reinforcement, and believe that additional exercise is unnecessary. Reasons often given for quitting exercise are inconvenience and lack of time. Several strategies have been suggested that can help you to increase and maintain your adherence to exercise. One method is to join an exercise program that has the following characteristics:

1. *Availability of program.* Change is facilitated by accessible programs. Find a program with convenient times and location.
2. *Social support.* It is important for you to include your family and/or "significant others" (i.e., persons important to you such as your spouse, work colleagues, or friends), so that they can encourage and support your participation in the fitness program.
3. *Emphasis on enjoyment.* Learning new behaviors must be pleasurable if you are to discard old behaviors. Choose an upbeat fitness program and activities that help you make fitness changes in an enjoyable atmosphere. The performance approach (e.g., military or athletic) aimed only at producing results while making you hate the exercise will *not* work in a lifelong fitness program. Think about the potential gains of your new behavior rather than any negative aspects. Your contract with a friend or helper should focus on these gains through activities you enjoy.
4. *Program attributes.* Qualified and enthusiastic personnel, regular assessment of important fitness components, relevant personal and general communication, and a variety of group/individual exercises, games, and sports that interest you are all qualities of a good fitness program. Physical exercise and socialization make a profitable combination, as evidenced by the success of many dance and physical fitness groups. Many people enjoy the social interaction with others, and a support group develops to help everyone continue the exercise.
5. *Role models.* People learn from each other and from others they admire. Choose a fitness instructor who displays healthy behaviors and enjoys a healthy lifestyle.

Another way to begin exercising is to do it on your own. In this case, signing a contract with a friend is a good way to begin. Table 14.2 shows an example of what such a contract might include. (Of course, you should modify it to be just right for you.)

## How Can I Stop Smoking?

There is little disagreement (outside cigarette-producing circles) that smoking is bad for health. There are ample data to show that smoking is the largest avoidable cause of death in the United States. Through warning labels on packages and in advertisements, virtually all U.S. citizens are now aware of smoking's dangers. Millions of people have quit smoking, but if you are a smoker, you know it is a difficult habit to break.

## Table 14.2
## Sample Contract to Begin Exercise

I, _____, do agree with _____ that I will begin the
  (your name)                                          (helper's name)

following walking program as of January 1, 1990:

1. I will walk from 7:00 to 7:30 A.M. on Monday, Wednesday, and Friday of each week.

2. I will record in writing my walking distance covered, and comments on a weekly form.

3. I will take this form to _____ each Sunday afternoon and discuss any problems
                                    (helper's name)
   I had as we walk together at 5:00 P.M.

4. In May, I will join the Plainview Fitness Center and attend a Tuesday/Thursday fitness class of my
   choice, continuing my Sunday afternoon walks with _____.
                                                            (helper's name)

I will reward myself with the purchase of one new record each week of perfect attendance in my program. At the end of each month of perfect attendance, I will buy a new compact disc of my choice. At the end of one year of perfect attendance, I will treat my helper and myself to a Broadway show in New York.

For each exercise session I miss, I will send a $25 contribution to the person who in my opinion is the most hypocritical politician.

_____        _____        _____
        (Signed)                       (Date)                     (Witness)

### Why Do I Smoke?

Remember, our first step in changing behavior is to analyze the problem. Perhaps a brief summary of some of the reasons people smoke will help you understand your own reasons. Many smokers start and continue the habit because they do it with friends or in certain situations. Others smoke while solving a problem, during a work break, watching a game, or after dinner. When do you smoke? Who else is around? What are you feeling when you smoke?

The so-called "rewards" of smoking include giving the smoker a series of "highs" when nicotine reaches the brain a few seconds after inhaling. An addiction to smoking is similar to addiction to other drugs. You experience a "craving" for a cigarette, and withdrawal symptoms make it a habit resistant to change. But you *can* break the habit, as millions have done. Now is a good time to do it.

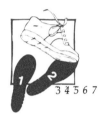

### What Is a Good Stop-Smoking Plan?

The following plan for stopping smoking includes: preparation, cessation, and maintenance.

***Stage 1: Preparation.*** You need to gain confidence that you can succeed in quitting smoking. Foster your self-confidence by setting clear goals and determining procedures to follow. During the first stage, you monitor your current frequency of smoking. This self-observation often helps to temporarily reduce your smoking behavior.

***Stage 2: Cessation.*** Ending the smoking behavior abruptly has been found to be more effective than gradually cutting down. An effective method to stop smoking is to sign a contract to quit on a specific date. The behavioral contract involves a specific agreement between you and another person. The goal is specified in terms of precise action. For example: "No cigarette will be smoked by Sheila Smith between the dates of December 31, 1989, and January 1, 1991." It is important that the behavior, or the lack of the behavior, be specifically described and linked to a time constraint. The contract also specifies the consequences if the contract is broken. For example, if Sheila Smith is a conservative Republican, her contract might stipulate that for each cigarette she smokes in 1989, she will send a $100 contribution to Senator Edward Kennedy of Massachusetts, a politician she particularly dislikes.

The contract should be individually tailored to your capabilities and needs. How long do you feel that you have to refrain from smoking to feel that you have quit? To whom can you send a donation to make the penalty especially aversive? What amount of money will help you abide by the conditions of the contract? Write into your contract any contingencies that will help you abide by the conditions of the contract. You will need frequent contact with your cosigner during the early part of the contract for encouragement and discussion of unanticipated problems. Table 14.3 outlines a sample contract that can be modified to fit your situation.

***Stage 3: Maintenance.*** Once again, an old joke makes a good point. The person says, "Stopping smoking is easy—I've done it hundreds of times!" The real problem, of course, is to find ways to keep from starting to smoke again once you have quit. Maintaining contact with your helper and developing new behavioral skills are essential ingredients in maintaining the behavioral change. Remind yourself of the advantages of a smokeless life (e.g., lower risk of major health problems, less stress in daily activities). You may have to learn

**Table 14.3**
# Sample Contract to Stop Smoking

I, _____, do agree with _____ to the following:
  (your name)                                    (helper's name)

1. Stop smoking as of 6:00 A.M., January 1, 1990.

2. I will call my helper each night at 7:00 P.M. during January, every Thursday night from February through May, and on the first of each month starting in June. We will discuss the problems I have had since our last call and set a time to meet if I need to talk with her in person.

3. During January, I will do the following at those times when, based on my past experience, I am most tempted to smoke:

   (a) Rub my pet rock with my right hand while talking with friends at social affairs

   (b) Eat fruit following dinner each night

   (c) Play a game of solitaire prior to going to sleep each night

I will reward myself with the purchase of one new record each week that I go without smoking. At the end of each smokeless month, I will buy a new compact disc of my choice. At the end of one year without smoking, I will treat my helper and myself to a Broadway show in New York.

For each cigarette I smoke during the year, I will send a $25 contribution to the person who in my opinion is the most hypocritical politician.

_____        _____        _____
      (Signed)                       (Date)                    (Witness)

new skills for dealing with old stimuli that you associate with cigarette smoking. If drinking coffee at the end of a meal was an old cue to light up, then perhaps avoiding coffee and drinking tea instead may eliminate that cue. If cigarette smoke in the lobby of a basketball arena during halftime provided a cue for lighting up, then either remaining seated in the arena or chewing gum in the lobby might be a new behavior. Once again we emphasize that determining what new behaviors you need and what will be effective often involves discussing your potential problem situations with others.

## How Can I Reduce Alcohol Consumption?

Alcoholism is one of our nation's leading public health problems. It is estimated that there are between 5 and 15 million alcoholics in the United States. The problems of family disruption, lost time at work, bodily injury, and death that are directly and indirectly due to excessive drinking are not disputed even by the producers of alcoholic beverages. The drinking problem exacts a heavy toll on the health and financial well-being of the people of the U.S.

Though there is no debate on the reality of the alcoholism problem, debate on appropriate goals for treating the problem is heated. Should an alcoholic strive for controlled moderate drinking or complete abstinence? Those who feel that abstinence is the correct goal tend to conceptualize the problem as a disease. The successful treatment approach of Alcoholics Anonymous (AA) is based on the disease concept. One fundamental precept of AA is that a person who has the disease of alcoholism will always have it—there is no cure. Combating the "disease" requires total abstinence. Alcoholics Anonymous helps individuals to achieve this goal with the support of other alcoholics via person-to-person contacts and regular group meetings.

Others contend that alcoholism is not a disease and that no crucial difference distinguishes the social drinker from the problem drinker besides the *amount* of alcohol consumed. Four factors that determine the probability of whether an individual will indulge in excessive drinking have been proposed: (a) the degree to which the individual feels controlled, (b) availability of an adequate coping response, (c) expectations about the results of the drinking, and (d) availability of alcohol and situational constraints. For example, (a) at a New Year's Eve party, you may feel strong pressure to drink; (b) you may

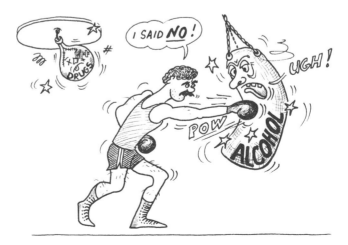

**Figure 14.2** Fighting addiction.

not have an adequate coping response—for example, you are unable to ask for a soft drink and request liquor instead; (c) you may have pleasant memories of previous New Year's Eve parties that included excessive drinking; and, (d) there is plenty of alcohol available, and party-goers are expected to consume it.

### Can I Control My Drinking?

If you believe that you can control your drinking, then several suggestions may help you. Social skills training to reduce excessive drinking normally includes instruction in assertive response, refusing alcohol, relapse prevention, and ways to obtain reinforcement other than from drinking. In assertiveness training you learn how to communicate your feelings in a productive, caring manner. This type of training may help you if your excessive drinking behavior is related to an inability to communicate feelings to intimates and other associates. Learning how to refuse alcoholic drinks is also important. Some alcoholics simply lack the cognitive awareness of verbalized sentences or words that they can use to refuse a drink. Learn and practice ways of refusing a drink.

Many techniques can enable you to abstain or drink less for a given period of time. However, it is difficult to maintain these improvements over a long period of time. Relapse prevention is probably the most important component of the social skills training plan. One of the key elements in maintaining the desired behavior is to be able to anticipate problem situations. Planning ways to avoid problems before the problems actually arise can help you discover behaviors other than excessive drinking that can provide positive reinforcement from your peers and important others. For example, improving your conversation or storytelling skills can give you a substitute for excessive drinking in some situations. You can use role-playing to avoid relapses. You need to learn to discuss your feelings and coping behaviors in potential problem situations with a helper.

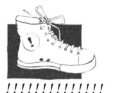

!!!!!!!!!!!!!!

### How Do I Choose Between Abstinence and Controlled Drinking?

You must decide which choice is appropriate for you. In general, someone with a history of chronic alcohol abuse who has developed serious life problems associated with drinking may be more suited to the complete abstinence approach. A younger person who is open to learning new social skills may respond well to the controlled drinking approach. A contract similar to the one for stopping smoking (Table 14.3) can be modified to help you either quit or control your drinking.

## How Can I Get to My Desired Weight?

Obesity seems to be more difficult to overcome than either smoking or problem drinking. Fewer than 5% of obese individuals successfully lose weight and maintain it whereas 20 to 25% report success at quitting smoking or alcohol abuse. One problem seems to be an emphasis on "negative change" goals rather than on developing healthy substitute behaviors. For example, instead of concentrating on eating less cheese, plan to eat fruit at snack time. Another problem is a disregard for either energy intake or energy expenditure. Both decreased caloric intake and increased exercise (caloric expenditure) are normally essential for maintaining desired weight. Either one by itself dooms most people to failure. Another problem is the direct attack on the behavior rather than on the indirect reasons for the behavior. If a particular cue results in poor eating behavior, then either avoid the cue or learn to react to it differently. The ready access of food and drink and media messages promoting a relationship between happiness and what you consume contribute to the problems for people trying to change their eating behaviors.

Chapter 4 dealt with methods of determining percent fat and estimating ideal weight. It is important that you work toward your goal gradually in ways that you can accept physiologically and psychologically.

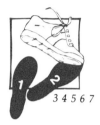

### How Can I Use a Weight Loss Program?

No single weight loss program can be recommended for all persons. The following seven components, however, appear to be common ingredients in all successful programs. Much of your success depends on you deciding what steps to take and what is likely to work for you to make it happen.

1. *Self-monitoring.* Before you implement any specific steps, keep a daily diary for 2 weeks. The diary should describe the quantity of food you eat and the eating environments.
2. *Treatment goals.* Once you determine your ideal weight goal, perhaps in consultation with a fitness leader, set weekly goals (from ½ to 2 pounds per week). If you are extremely obese (> 40% fat if female, > 30% fat if male), seek medical supervision.
3. *Diet selection.* Select a dietary plan that specifies food type, portions, and calorie amounts. You may want to use the Basic Four Food Group plan and the Exchange System outlined in chapter 5.
4. *Stimulus control.* Certain situations or cues are often strongly related to eating patterns (e.g., watching a movie or television). Decide to eat only at certain places (e.g., the dining room table, the cafeteria at work) only at certain times (e.g., breakfast, lunch, supper, and one snack time).
5. *Self-reward.* Some people are helped by giving themselves small rewards for progress toward their goals (e.g., a new audio tape for each 3-pound loss) and a larger reward (e.g., tickets to a Broadway show) when they reach the final goal. The rewards should be consistent with healthy behaviors, something you enjoy, and things for which there are no acceptable alternatives.
6. *Exercise.* The first section of this chapter dealt with ways to begin and continue regular exercise. Although everyone who begins an exercise program does not necessarily need to begin a diet reduction program, most people who need to lose fat should begin diet and exercise programs simultaneously.
7. *Support.* The awareness and support of a spouse or other important person can greatly assist you in staying with the program. The involvement of friends or family members early in the program enhances the probability of its success.

## How Can I Reduce Stress?

Attempts to understand human stress (see chapter 10) and to develop plans to alleviate it are relatively recent. We recommend that you pay attention to

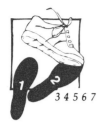

your interaction with potential stressors as a way to reduce excessive stress. You can go through the suggested steps by yourself, but you may find it helpful to work with a fitness leader or counselor.

Three stages of stress reduction are preparation, skill acquisition, and practice.

1. In the first stage, you prepare yourself mentally for a coming stressful situation. Keep a diary regarding the frequency of and conditions surrounding the chosen stressor.

2. In the skill acquisition stage, the main emphasis is on learning basic cognitive and behavioral coping skills. One of the skills is "private speech," where you learn sentences to say to yourself prior to, during, and following the stressor. For example, prior to a major test or presentation of a report tell yourself, "Its going to be hard, but I have prepared for it." During the event: "If I stay calm I will be less likely to block on a question," and/or "I'm getting tense—relax and take it easy." Following the event: "I did as well as I could because I stayed calm."

    A second component of the skill acquisition stage is relaxation training. Chapter 10 outlined a procedure of tensing and relaxing specific muscle groups. With practice, you can rapidly achieve a relaxed state in a potentially stressful situation.

3. In the final, or practice, stage, you set up a series of practice situations that help you learn to apply the previously taught skills. The sequence of situations progresses from relatively mild to more severe stress so that you can experience success and gain confidence in using the skills.

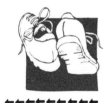

## Summary

One of the primary responsibilities of a fitness program is to help participants modify lifestyle behaviors. Although the focus of attention is on increasing exercise, it should be clear that unhealthy behaviors need to be decreased. These behaviors include smoking, excessive alcohol consumption, overeating, and stress. Each of these behaviors is discussed in terms of what causes them and the methods you can use to change the specific behavior. Some commonalities exist among the behavior change techniques. These guidelines can help you change behavior: If you desire to change a behavior, analyze the history of the problem and record the current status of the behavior. Set a long-term goal and several short-term goals, and sign a contract with a friend. List as many strategies as possible to resolve the problem, selecting one or two that will be most effective. Learn new coping skills and have regular meetings with a helper. Once you reach the goal, outline a maintenance schedule that includes periodic contacts with your helper.

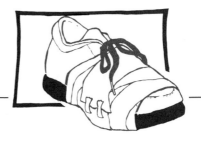

## Chapter
## *15*

# *How Can I Prevent and Deal With Injury?*

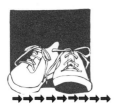

| |
|---|
| **How Can I Avoid Injury?** |
| **What Should I Do If I Injure Myself?** |
| **How Do I Deal With Specific Orthopedic Problems?** |
| **What About Emergencies?** |
| **What Are the Risks of Injury?** |

When you cross the street, drive a car, operate a lawn mower, or climb a ladder you are risking injury. If even these common tasks have a risk of injury, it should be no surprise that participation in a physical activity program, even one related to improving health status, is not without risks as well.

## What Are the Risks of Injury?

There is good evidence that the risk of injury increases for workouts conducted at intensities greater than 85% maximal heart rate, durations longer than 40 minutes, and frequencies greater than four times per week. Activities such as running and exercise to music cause more muscle and skeletal trauma than riding a stationary cycle or swimming. Games, especially competitive ones, are associated with more injuries than are controlled, low-intensity, cooperative games.

However, the potential for injury goes beyond the type, intensity, frequency, and duration of activity. The environment and the characteristics of the participant also contribute to overall injury risk. Exercising in a hot, humid environment predisposes you to heat injury, while exercising in the cold can lead to frostbite and hypothermia. Not surprisingly, older, less fit individuals are more susceptible to skeletal injuries than are young, fit people. Finally, someone with a medical condition such as asthma or diabetes requires special attention to avoid a situation that could result in serious trouble. The purpose of all this is not to scare you to the point of not participating in an exercise program; rather, we wish to set forth issues that you must address to minimize the risks associated with exercise programs.

## How Can I Minimize Injury Risk?

As we have indicated throughout the preceding chapters, one of the most important things to do to minimize risk is to undergo a health screening before beginning an exercise program. On the basis of the screening you may be referred for additional tests, placed in a medically supervised program, or told that exercising in a graduated program like the one described in chapter 11 represents a low risk. Our recommended exercise program focuses attention on starting slowly, progressing in an orderly fashion from low to moderate intensities, and avoiding more uncontrolled activities until you achieve a solid fitness base. It is important to listen to your body, pay attention to signals that indicate you may be doing too much, and slow down (see Figure 15.1). Even if you heed this advice, however, you may still experience an injury during exercise. Therefore we must move beyond these recommendations and discuss the treatment of common injuries associated with exercise.

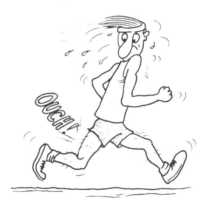

**Figure 15.1** Listen to your body.

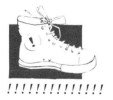

One of the most common problems associated with starting an exercise program is muscle soreness. It is important to understand that muscle soreness is a normal sensation associated with any new physical activity.

If you are an avid jogger who puts in 12 miles a week and decide to participate in a game of soccer, which emphasizes sudden bursts of speed, changes of direction, and explosive kicks, don't be surprised by the muscle soreness that shows up 24 to 48 hours after the game. The soreness is related to actual tissue damage in the active muscles and the inflammation response (swelling) that follows. Once you have experienced soreness, it usually does not recur in those muscles as a result of the same activity unless a long period of time (6 to 9 weeks) elapses between exposures. The following signs and symptoms associated with injury are listed here to call your attention to circumstances that may require some special attention. If you experience them, we encourage you to discuss them with your fitness instructor and physician. Though these signs and symptoms can also appear in an extreme case of muscle soreness, in general that is not the case.

### Signs of Injury

1. Extreme tenderness when body part is touched
2. Pain while at rest; pain that will not disappear after warming up; joint pain; increased pain when moving or exercising that body part
3. Swelling or discoloration
4. Changes in normal body function

## What Is the Best Treatment for Common Injuries?

The most common injuries associated with exercise programs are sprains and strains. Sprains are caused by the stretching of the connective tissue (ligaments) surrounding a joint, while strains occur when muscles or tendons are stretched. Figure 15.2 shows that the immediate treatment of both conditions is summed up by the acronym *PRICE*, which stands for *Protecting* and *Resting* the injured body part and using *Ice* with *Compression* on the body part, which should be *Elevated* to reduce fluid accumulation.

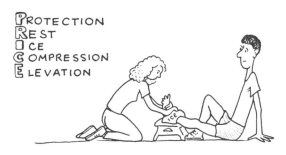

**Figure 15.2**  The PRICE is right.

The steps described below will tend to reduce the swelling associated with an injury and reduce the time needed for normal function to return. Ice helps to reduce the blood flow to the injured site as well as the sensation of pain. Follow this same set of steps when a muscle is damaged by a direct blow (contusion), or when the heel of the foot strikes a hard surface, causing a "stone bruise." In the case of a contusion the muscle should usually be stretched before the ice is applied, and a soft pad should be placed under the heel to reduce the force of impact for a heel bruise.

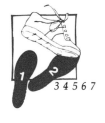

### Immediate Treatment of Common Injuries

1. *Protect* the body part from further damage.
2. *Rest* the body part; do not try to "walk it off."
3. *Ice* (crushed or cubes in a plastic bag) is applied for 20 to 30 minutes and is repeated on a regular basis—hourly, or when pain occurs. Ice treatment should continue for 24 to 72 hours depending on the degree of injury.
4. *Compression* bandages should be used to hold the ice bag in place and also when the ice is removed. The bandage is wrapped firmly, but not too tightly, to help minimize swelling.
5. *Elevate* the injured body part whenever possible.

Moderate injuries (exhibiting swelling, discoloration, and joint tenderness) to severe injuries (exhibiting extreme tenderness and swelling, discoloration, and deformity of body part) should be examined by a physician. Always remember to follow the PRICE steps for any acute (recent) injury. You may apply heat later in the recovery process when the swelling and the chance of more bleeding (which causes more swelling) are reduced. In addition, people with chronic problems like tendonitis or bursitis, may apply heat prior to activity. If you are ever in doubt, use ice.

# How Do I Deal With Common Orthopedic Problems?

A number of orthopedic problems have a common denominator: overuse. Skeletal muscles, connective tissue (both tendons and ligaments), and tissues in or around joints can be affected. We do not mean that overuse is the only cause of orthopedic problems; infection and direct physical trauma can also cause them. The following is a brief list of common conditions:

- **Bursitis**   Inflammation of the bursa, which is a fluid-filled sac between muscle and bone that aids in movement
- **Tendonitis**   Inflammation of a tendon, which is the tissue tying a muscle to a bone
- **Myositis**   Inflammation of a muscle
- **Synovitis**   Inflammation of the synovial membrane, which forms the inner lining of joint cavities and secretes synovial fluid to aid in the movement of the bones in the joint space
- **Plantar Fasciitis**   Inflammation of the connective tissue on the bottom of the foot

The constant in all of these definitions is the process of *inflammation*, which is the body's normal reaction to infection or trauma. Tennis elbow and shin splints (more on these later) are examples of inflammatory reactions involving muscles and connective tissue. Inflammation involves special white blood cells as well as chemicals that increase the pores in capillaries to let large proteins enter the injured area. This influx of protein brings water along, causing the swelling.

### How Do I Treat Overuse Problems?

The immediate treatment for these problems is the same as for sprains: ice and rest. If the problem is a chronic (long-term) one, warming the area before physical activity and using ice afterward can help reduce pain and discomfort. An obvious recommendation is to stop doing the activity that causes the problem and shift to another activity. For joggers who develop problems with their knees, swimming is a good substitute. For swimmers who develop shoulder problems, cycling is a good substitute. Have your physician examine any chronic inflammatory condition that limits your normal daily function.

*Stress fractures* to the lower leg and the foot are also caused by overuse. This problem occurs when the bone's ability to adapt to a chronic load is exceeded. The area over the fracture is very tender to the touch. Pain is present most of the time but increases when you stand. Stress fractures need physician care and take a long time to heal (6 to 10 weeks). Any supplemental exercises you use during the recovery process must be approved by your physician.

### What About Shin Splints?

Shin splints refer to an inflammation of the muscle-tendon unit on the front side of the lower leg. This injury has a wide variety of causes, including overuse. It is more common to runners and dancers (including participants in exercise-to-music programs) because of the special load these participants place on the lower leg during exercise. However, weak arches, hard surfaces, inadequate shoes, structural abnormalities, and improper exercise techniques can all cause shin splints. Needless to say, the recommended ways to deal with this injury are as varied as the list of causes.

- **Overuse** Cut back on the total amount of running or dancing, or simply substitute something else.
- **Surface** Running or dancing on softer surfaces will help absorb the shock of impact.
- **Shoes** Well-cushioned and properly designed exercise shoes will help to dissipate the shock of impact.

Don't be fooled into believing that the simple purchase of an excellent (and expensive!) pair of exercise shoes will make shin splints disappear. Shoes can help reduce the problem, but you must also exercise good judgment about the overuse issue. Some people use their good shoes and soft floor as a rationale to do even more exercise, resulting in an aggravation of the problem. Add variety to your workout to reduce the chance that you will overstress any single area of your body.

## How Do I Modify Exercise to Make It Safer?

Table 15.1 on page 142 summarizes the classifications of injury with the terms *mild, moderate,* and *severe,* and offers some suggestions on how to deal with them. Please recognize that this list is *not* a prescription to follow. If you hear a "pop," feel a deformity, or think you have a serious injury, contact a physician. For those injuries you believe to be mild, we suggest you find activities that minimize the role of the injured part. Often you can use water or cycling (with legs or arms) exercises that do not affect the injury. In some cases, you may have to refrain from your usual exercise until the injury is better. If your own exercise modifications do not result in a relief of the problem after 2 to 4 weeks, consult a physician. When the injured part gets better, do very light exercises involving that part and gradually increase the exercise intensity. Avoid quick movements of the injured part. Trying to do too much too soon after an injury often results in reinjury.

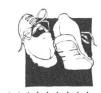

## Summary

The risk of injury associated with physical activity increases for workouts conducted in excess of 85% of maximal heart rate, durations longer than 40 minutes, and frequencies greater than four times per week. Risks are greater in competitive games compared to stationary cycling, and for older, less fit persons compared to younger, more fit individuals. The risk of injury is minimized by participation in a screening prior to an exercise program, starting at low levels, progressing in small steps, and developing a fitness base before engaging in less controlled activities. It is important to distinguish simple

**Table 15.1**
**Criteria for Assessing Severity of Injury and Suggested Exercise Modifications**

| Criteria | Modifications |
| --- | --- |
| *Mild Injury* | |
| 1. Performance not affected | 1. Reduce activity level |
| 2. Pain experienced only after athletic activity | 2. Modify activity to take stress off of the injured part |
| 3. Generally, no tenderness on palpation | 3. Symptomatic treatment |
| 4. No or minimal swelling | 4. Gradual return to full activity |
| 5. No discoloration | |
| *Moderate Injury* | |
| 1. Performance mildly affected or not affected at all | 1. Rest the injured part |
| 2. Pain experienced before and after athletic activity | 2. Modify activity to take stress off of the injured part |
| 3. Mild tenderness on palpation | 3. Symptomatic treatment |
| 4. Mild swelling may be present | 4. Gradual return to full activity |
| 5. Some discoloration may be present | |
| *Severe Injury* | |
| 1. Pain experienced before, during, and after activity | 1. Complete rest |
| 2. Performance definitely affected because of pain | 2. Referral to a physician |
| 3. Normal daily function affected because of pain | |
| 4. Movement limited because of pain | |
| 5. Moderate to severe point tenderness on palpation | |
| 6. Swelling most likely present | |
| 7. Discoloration may be present | |

*Note.* From Howley and Franks (1986).

muscle soreness from serious injury. Acute injuries, including sprains, strains, contusions, and bone bruises shoud be treated with the PRICE approach: Protect and Rest the injured part, use Ice with Compression, and Elevate the injured part. Besides strains and sprains, most common orthopedic problems are inflammation reactions caused by overuse. The treatment of an acute inflammation includes ice and rest, similar to the treatment for a sprain. For chronic problems, however, you may warm the inflamed area before a workout to help relieve discomfort during the activity and use the ice treatment after the workout. A better choice is to change activities to rest the injured area. If your daily function is limited by such inflammation injuries, consult a physician. Shin splints is a condition affecting the front part of the lower leg and is found primarily in runners and dance-exercisers. The condition is relieved by changing activities, decreasing the intensity/duration of the current activity, and using well-cushioned surfaces and shoes.

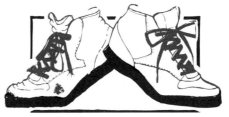

# Chapter
# 16

# What About Special Personal or Medical Conditions?

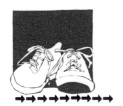

---

**How Do I Make Fitness Changes With**
   **Physical Conditions?**
   **Medical Conditions?**

---

If you develop an injury or have a special medical condition, you really need to modify your exercise program or use special caution in planning it. The following sections of this chapter outline only a few of the problems that may need attention. Please use good judgment in your approach to exercise; if you experience new pains or strange sensations it is wise to have these checked out before continuing with your exercise program.

## What if I Have Health or Physical Problems?

### Orthopedic Problems

If you have pain in the ankle, knee, or hip when you walk or jog, cut back on the amount of activity that you are doing or change the activity itself. For example, a jogger can switch to swimming or cycling to take a load off the ankle, knee, or hip. If you have a chronic orthopedic problem, choose an activity that will not aggravate it. In addition, you might follow the recommendations in chapter 15 about how to deal with chronic inflammation problems. Generally, it is important to do a long warm-up and use ice afterward to minimize any swelling that may occur. Again, seriously consider an alternate activity that will take a load off the joints that are bothering you. If the condition persists for several weeks, see a physician.

## Diabetes

If you or someone you know has diabetes, special attention must be paid to diet and medication (if any is taken) when exercising. An insulin-dependent diabetic should discuss any planned exercise program with a physician or nurse-educator to deal properly *and safely* with special considerations. An insulin-dependent diabetic has to achieve good "control" (a near-normal blood glucose concentration) by varying diet and insulin. Exercise complicates this balancing act in that exercise usually increases the rate at which glucose is removed from the blood, necessitating a reduction of the insulin dose or an increase in carbohydrate intake before exercise. However, for the insulin-dependent diabetic who has an extremely elevated glucose level before exercise, the activity may actually cause a further increase in the blood glucose and the development of ketosis, pushing the diabetic further out of control. Consequently, it is necessary for the insulin-dependent diabetic to develop good control before starting an exercise program and to maintain a careful and systematic approach to exercise. The vast majority of insulin-dependent diabetics can do this, and we encourage it. Exercise allows the diabetic to have a normal, active lifestyle. Special attention must be paid to the insulin dose; too much will cause dangerous hypoglycemia (low blood glucose), and too little results in worsening control over blood glucose. Remember, control is the most important goal for an insulin-dependent diabetic. Carbohydrate intake may have to be increased before exercise to meet the greater need that the exercise will cause. After exercise additional carbohydrate will be needed to replace what was used from muscle stores. As always, frequent monitoring of blood glucose is the best way to keep tabs on this balancing act.

Only 10% of all diabetics are insulin-dependent. The rest are classified as adult-onset diabetics. This form of diabetes generally occurs after the age of 40 and it is associated with obesity. This diabetic usually produces a sufficient amount of insulin, but the tissues are simply resistant to it. Although oral medication may be taken to stimulate the production of more insulin, most of these diabetics are treated simply with diet and exercise to achieve weight loss and help normalize blood glucose. Exercise makes the person less resistant to insulin so that the available insulin may be sufficient to meet the body's needs. In fact, some diabetics may have to cut back or stop their intake of oral medication as a result of their exercise programs. In addition, the combination of diet and exercise can result in a weight loss that causes the condition to disappear. Follow these guidelines when planning an exercise program:

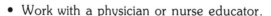

- Work with a physician or nurse educator.
- Adjust medication (if taking any) prior to exercise.
- Increase carbohydrate intake if needed.
- Inform the exercise leader that you are a diabetic.
- Carry along a readily available form of glucose in case of hypoglycemia.
- Exercise with a "buddy" who can help out in an emergency.

## Asthma

Asthma is a condition in which the airways suddenly reduce in size, making it difficult to breathe. This condition can be caused by a wide variety of environmental factors, such as pollen and pollutants, in susceptible individuals. Exercise itself may trigger asthma attacks in some people. This condition, called *exercise-induced asthma*, is brought on by breathing great volumes of air that dries and cools the respiratory tract. This causes a series of changes, including a constriction of the airway and an increased secretion of fluid into the airway. It is a frightening experience, but there is little question that it can be controlled. Sixty-seven athletes in the 1984 Olympic Games had this problem, and 41 of them won medals! The problem is controlled by medications taken prior to exercise that prevent the condition from occurring. This is the recommended course of action, and it is important enough that a concerned exercise leader should ask if an affected individual has taken the medication (see Figure 16.1).

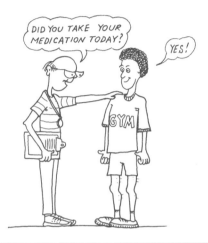

**Figure 16.1**  Take medication as prescribed.

For those who are sensitive to the problem, we recommend a long warm-up period prior to strenuous exercise, and the exercise should be done in periods of 5 minutes or less. Because breathing warm, moist air reduces the chance of an attack, swimming is a recommended activity for persons in this group. Runners and cyclists can reduce drying of the respiratory passages by wearing a scarf or mask that may trap some of the moisture. An asthmatic should take along an aerosol bronchodilator in case the wheezing starts during exercise. Here are some guidelines to follow:

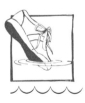

- Work with your physician to control the asthma with medication.
- Take medication prior to exercise.
- Do a long warm-up and short-interval activities.
- Inform the exercise leader that you have asthma.
- Carry along an aerosol bronchodilator.
- Exercise with a "buddy" who can help out in an emergency.

## Obesity

Exercise is a normal part of a weight loss program for obese or overweight individuals. In general, the recommended pattern of weight loss includes dividing the caloric deficit between dietary reduction and exercise to about 50:50 or 60:40, respectively. The overweight individual has probably been sedentary for some period of time; we recommend the walking program as the best place to start. Walking can be done each day and in all kinds of weather so that daily or weekly energy expenditure is predictable. As weight is lost fewer calories are expended per mile of walking and the distance will have to be increased slightly to compensate for that. The idea is to get the overweight person moving into a regular pattern of activity with the lowest probability of injury. Walking fills the bill. However, for people with joint problems, swimming and cycling are excellent alternatives to consider.

### High Blood Pressure

Hypertension is a very common problem in our country and one that needs to be controlled to reduce the chance of heart attacks and strokes. We recommend that you have your blood pressure checked on a regular basis, and if it is elevated, see a physician. The physician may recommend medications as well as changes in diet (especially sodium), weight loss, and/or exercise. The important thing is to get the blood pressure under control. The recommended exercise programs outlined in chapters 11 and 12 are the kinds of activities that have been used successfully in hypertensive populations. The emphasis is on large muscle activity done in a dynamic fashion. Small muscle activities or those requiring a breath hold tend to increase blood pressure and should be avoided. If you are hypertensive, it is important to remember to take whatever medication has been prescribed at the same time each day. In this way, if blood pressure is monitored prior to an exercise class, you will receive good feedback about how close to normal you are maintaining the pressure. In addition, because diet, weight loss, and exercise can in themselves cause a reduction in pressure, the blood pressure reading acts as a signal of when it is time to return to the physician for a change or elimination of medication.

One major type of blood pressure medication is the diuretic, which causes a loss of sodium and water from the body. If you are on this type of medication while exercising, you must be careful to maintain an adequate fluid intake. The sweat associated with exercise results in an additional loss of sodium and water from your body. This could result in a lower blood pressure than is desirable. If you are taking a beta adrenergic blocking agent (e.g., Inderal® ) to control blood pressure, you should not use the formula (220 − age) for calculating the maximal heart rate. This medication lowers the maximal heart rate, and your usual THR zone calculation will be incorrect. Work with your physician and fitness professional to determine the appropriate THR zone if you are on medication. The following steps are recommended for a hypertensive person:

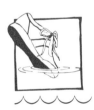

- Work with your physician to control the hypertension.
- If medication is prescribed, take it regularly.
- Do dynamic activities involving large muscle groups.
- Have your blood pressure measured regularly.

### Seizure Disorders

Like the diabetic and the asthmatic, a person with a controlled seizure disorder (like epilepsy) is encouraged to participate in a regular physical activity program and lead a normal life. If you have a seizure disorder we recommend that you inform your exercise leader about the condition. If you exercise away from a group, exercise with a "buddy" who can provide assistance in case of an emergency. Further, do not jog alone near traffic or swim in an unsupervised pool. We recommend the following steps if you have a seizure disorder:

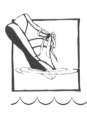

- Take your prescribed medication regularly.
- Inform your exercise leader about your condition.
- Exercise with a "buddy".

### Age-Associated Problems

In our discussions on exercise, we have focused on maintaining cardio-respiratory fitness. This applies to the elderly as well, but exercise also helps this group to maintain the mineral content of bone and control osteoporosis, a thinning of bone that increases the chance of fracture. Exercise acts along with calcium and hormones to maintain the integrity of the bones. The following classification of the elderly was proposed by researchers Smith and Gilligan in 1987:

- **Athletic old** > 55 years with good fitness (10 METs)
- **Young old** > 55 years with moderate fitness (6 to 7 METs)
- **Old old** > 75 years with very low fitness (2 to 3 METs)

Our exercise recommendations vary rather dramatically with this group. The athletic old can do the program described in chapter 12 with few modifications. The young old have the fitness level of cardiac patients and are therefore limited in their choice of activities. However, walking, cycling, and swimming at low intensities are well within their capability and are to be encouraged. The old old group is extremely limited in choice, and the vast majority of fitness activities are done with the person lying, sitting, or standing with support.

It is important for everyone to be active. However, the older and more at risk an individual is from osteoporosis, the greater the need for controlled activities that will not result in fracture. Activities such as walking, cycling, and swimming all fit the bill. However, the upward posture associated with walking appears to place special and appropriate stress on the bones due to the force of gravity, making walking the primary recommended activity for older people.

## Pregnancy

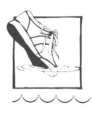

Women are encouraged to stay active when they become pregnant. Just like the diabetic or the asthmatic, the pregnant woman should discuss any exercise plans with her physician, as the fetus already places an additional burden on a woman's systems. Exercise does not appear to deprive the fetus of oxygen, and the fetus's heart rate shows no signs of distress during exercise. Compared to the exercise guidelines established for cardiac patients, those for pregnant women are gradually developing. Although some physicians suggest that a pregnant woman should not begin an exercise program, others believe that moderate exercise conducted on a regular basis is a reasonable goal for those interested. The guidelines from the American College of Obstetricians and Gynecologists include the following:

- Work with your physician to plan the exercise program.
- Follow a 3-day-per-week pattern, with warm-up and cool-down.
- Avoid intense activities causing heart rate above 140 beats per minute.
- Avoid prolonged activity or activity in hot, humid weather that can raise body temperature above 100.4 °F.
- Do not perform exercises while lying on your back after the 4th month of pregnancy.
- Avoid ballistic movements and deep flexion and extension exercises.

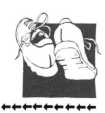

## Summary

Many health problems or personal characteristics influence the kinds of activity you can do in a fitness program. This chapter provided some suggestions to assist you, as you work with your physician, in selecting appropriate exercises to use with orthopedic problems, diabetes, asthma, obesity, high blood pressure, seizure disorders, aging, and pregnancy. General recommendations for anyone who has questions about exercise are to check with a personal physician; use longer warm-ups; slow the progression to the main part of the workout; lower the intensity of the activity; use longer cool-down activities; pay attention to environmental conditions; recognize signs of overexertion; exercise with others; be regular with food, water, and prescribed medication; and use common sense in deciding to modify or stop an activity.

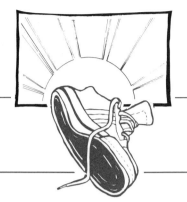

## Chapter
## 17

# What About Environmental Conditions?

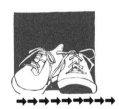

→→→→→→→→→

---

### How Do I Exercise in Different Environments?

---

The emphasis in our recommended exercise program is on safety, so that fitness gains are made with minimal risk. We use THR as a means of setting a level of intensity that allows an adequate duration of exercise for a fitness effect and expends a reasonable number of calories.

## How Do Different Environments Affect My Exercise?

Unfortunately, factors besides exercise can affect your heart rate response and your ability to complete a workout. The information we present here deals with these factors and suggests some ways to alter your workout.

### How Do Heat and Humidity Affect Exercise?

Your body temperature increases with exercise due to the heat the muscles produce, and it usually stabilizes at a safe level as heat loss catches up and equals the rate of heat production. This balance can be upset if your body (a) gains too much heat from the environment and/or (b) is unable to evaporate enough sweat to get rid of the heat. If the environmental temperature (outdoors or indoors) is higher than skin temperature, you actually gain heat from the air rather than lose heat to it. This heat load causes higher than usual body temperature and heart rate responses. In this situation, evaporation of sweat from the skin becomes the primary means of heat loss. The ideal environment has low relative humidity that increases evaporation of sweat, reducing body heat. The higher the relative humidity, the more difficult it is for sweat to evaporate; this also drives up body temperature and heart rate. When the body cannot adequately handle the heat load, a variety of problems, classified as heat injuries, can occur. These are listed below, from least to most dangerous:

---

### Heat Injuries

| Classification | Signs and symptoms |
|---|---|
| 1. **Heat syncope:** | **Headaches, nausea, light-headedness** |
| 2. **Muscle cramps:** | **Spasms in muscle; more dangerous when more than one muscle is affected** |
| 3. **Heat exhaustion:** | **Lots of sweating, cold and clammy skin, pale skin, dizziness, nausea, headache, loss of consciousness** |
| 4. **Heat stroke:** | **No sweating, hot and dry skin, extremely high body temperature, rapid and strong pulse** |

---

It is important that you attend to the following signs and symptoms that may indicate trouble:

- Hair standing on end on arms, back, and chest
- Chills
- Throbbing in the head, or headache
- Vomiting or nausea
- Dry lips or "cotton mouth"
- Muscle cramping
- Light-headedness
- No sweating

You must be aware of these signs and symptoms and, if they occur, act on them immediately. If you feel light-headed and experience nausea, stop, get to a cool place, sit or lie down with your feet elevated, and drink some fluids. Treat a muscle cramp by putting direct pressure on the muscle, massaging it, and stretching it gently. If you experience multiple cramps or the symptoms of heat exhaustion, go to a cool place, lie down with your feet up, drink lots of fluids, and see a physician when you feel better. Heat stroke is treated as a medical emergency—get to a hospital as soon as possible, remove clothing, and cool down starting at the head with ice, cold wet towels, fans, and so on.

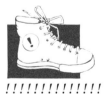

!!!!!!!!!!!!!!!

***Prevention of Heat Injury.*** The message is clear: When you exercise in an environment with high heat and humidity, you must decrease the normal intensity of your exercise to keep your heart rate from going too high, whether you are indoors or outdoors. How do you do this? Simply *monitor your pulse rate* during the exercise session, and when you find it to be near the *top part of the THR* zone, *decrease the intensity* of exercise.

Prevention is always better than treatment; this is especially true of heat injuries. Prevention demands that you be aware of both sides of the heat gain/heat loss equation. When the environmental temperature is higher than skin temperature, you will gain heat from the environment in addition to what your muscles are producing. This is not a problem if (a) the air is "dry" enough to allow evaporation of enough sweat to compensate for this heat gain, and (b) the body can produce necessary sweat. Let's look at each of these conditions.

*Evaporation.*  All of us have had the *experience* of doing exercise or physical labor when the temperature has been in the 90s but we did not feel too uncomfortable. On another day, with the same high temperature, the work might have been unbearable. Why? In the first case the relative humidity was probably low. The air contained very little moisture, making it *easy* for sweat to evaporate from skin and keep the body cool. When the relative humidity is high, sweat simply runs down into our socks and does not evaporate. If sweat does not evaporate, body heat cannot be lost and body temperature rises.

Another issue related to your ability to evaporate sweat is that sweat must get to the surface of the body before it can be evaporated. We still see advertisements for special workout suits ("sauna suits") that claim to help you lose weight when you exercise. These suits are made of plastic, rubber, or nylon material that is impermeable to sweat. The result is that sweat does not evaporate, and body temperature increases. This can be dangerous. The extra body weight lost with such procedures is all water weight that *must* be replaced before your next workout. The best recommendation is to wear as little clothing as possible. It is important to expose as much skin as you dare (e.g., wear mesh fabrics) to allow sweat to evaporate. Cotton clothing is good because it "wicks" sweat to its surface.

*Sweat.*  Assuming that the environment is conducive to the evaporation of sweat and that you are wearing the proper clothing, how can you be sure that you will be able to sweat enough to lose the heat? You can do several things to improve your chances. One of the most important is to allow yourself to adjust *gradually* to the heat and humidity over a period of 7 to 10 days. This means that you should ease into your exercise program during the coolest part of the day, gradually shifting the workout to the warmer part of the day. As you spend more and more time in the heat and humidity, your body begins to sweat *more* (not less), improving the chance that you will be able to maintain your body temperature in the safe zone. In spite of the increased sweat rate, you will lose no more salt from the body than you did before because the body learns to hold onto more of its salt. If you are sweating more, it logically follows that you must drink more water.

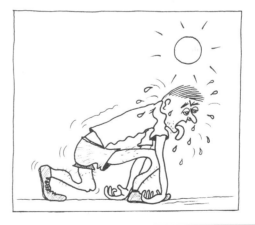

**Figure 17.1**  Did you drink enough water today?

*Guidelines for Salt and Water Replacement.*  It is very important that you be in water balance (i.e., have the proper amount of body water) prior to a workout. Drink water *before*, *during*, and *after* the activity. It is difficult for the body to sweat fast enough to get rid of the heat if there is not enough water to produce the sweat. One of the best ways to see if you have been drinking enough water is to weigh yourself before each workout. If you have lost two pounds between workouts, that is equal to being a "quart low" on water. If you drink too much water you will simply urinate the excess. Cold water (40-60 °F) is absorbed faster than warm water, but independent of temperature, make sure you get your fill. More is better than less.

This, however, does not hold true for salt. Sweat is a very dilute salt solution—the body loses more water than salt during exercise. This is why it is more important to replace the water. Salt can be replaced at mealtime, and in our country most of us take in more salt than we need. Do not use salt tablets. If you feel you need additional salt, simply shake more salt on your food at your next mealtime.

Are commercially available electrolyte drinks (e.g., Gatorade) a better way to replace fluid lost in exercise? Generally, plain old water is all you need to replace the water lost in sweat. In fact, some electrolyte drinks contain so much sugar they are actually absorbed slower than water. The salt and other minerals lost in sweat are adequately replaced at mealtime.

The following is a set of guidelines regarding exercise in heat and humidity:

- Don't exercise in environments that will not allow heat loss.
- When very hot, humid weather is forecast, choose a cooler part of the day to exercise.
- Gradually increase your exposure to the heat and humidity over a period of 7 to 10 days.
- Wear clothing that facilitates the evaporation of sweat.
- *Use your THR as a guide to change the intensity of the exercise.*
- Drink extra water before exercise, drink during exercise, and replace what you have lost after exercise.
- If you must, use additional salt at mealtime. Do not take salt tablets.
- If you feel light-headed, nauseated, or flushed, stop exercising, get out of the heat, drink water, and cool down with wet cloths, fans, and so forth.

### Should I Be Concerned About Exercising in the Cold?

Exercising in the cold can be refreshing, but it can also be dangerous. You must be ready to treat cold with the same amount of precaution that you did heat. Cold air causes the blood vessels in the skin to constrict to prevent warm blood from giving up its heat to the environment. This is good because body temperature is protected. However, the constriction, if pronounced and prolonged, can lead to frostbite. In addition, cold air may cause susceptible individuals to experience angina (chest pain) or an asthma attack. Regard windchill temperatures lower than −20 °F as a frostbite alert, and pay attention to the increased possibility of irritation of the respiratory tract. You may choose to deal with such circumstances by not exercising in extremely cold temperatures, or simply by doing your workout indoors. Because there are so many available health club facilities that offer comprehensive exercise programs as well as shopping malls to use as walking trails, people have learned how to work around this problem. If frostbite does occur, immerse the affected body part in warm water without massaging.

The major concern about exercising in cold weather relates to the condition of *hypothermia*, which simply means losing body heat faster than it is produced. This leads to a decrease in body temperature that can trigger violent shivering, impair neuromuscular function (balance, the ability to do things, speech), decrease the ability to make decisions, and make you feel so tired that you must rest. The problem, of course, is that if you decide to rest in the cold you will die! Interestingly, hypothermia occurs frequently in temperatures above 30 °F. If an individual is exercising in such cold conditions and produces a great deal of sweat, the sweat evaporates very quickly because cold air is dry. This causes the loss of body heat. If a person is exercising in cold, rainy weather, the moisture on the surface of the skin evaporates like sweat, causing an additional heat loss.

If you have the unfortunate experience of falling into cold water, get out quickly. Heat is lost from the body about 20 times faster in water compared to air at the same temperature.

An additional factor related to heat loss in the cold is *windchill* (Table 17.1). This term refers to the fact that the temperature we experience at the skin is lower than the actual air temperature when the wind is blowing. As the cold (dry) air passes by the skin, heat is lost directly to the air, and the dry air increases the evaporation of moisture from the skin. When you plan a workout, consider the fact that if you ride a bicycle at 15 miles per hour into cold *still* air you will experience a temperature much lower than the air temperature indicates.

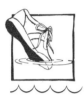

The best way to deal with hypothermia is to prevent its occurrence. Here is a list of suggestions to that end:

- Do not exercise in extreme cold and wind; use indoor activities.
- Wear layers of clothing; remove layers as you warm up.
- Stay as dry as possible.

**Table 17.1**
**Wind Chill Index**

| Wind speed in MPH | Actual thermometer reading (°F) | | | | | | | | | | | |
|---|---|---|---|---|---|---|---|---|---|---|---|---|
| | 50 | 40 | 30 | 20 | 10 | 0 | −10 | −20 | −30 | −40 | −50 | −60 |
| | Equivalent temperature (°F) | | | | | | | | | | | |
| Calm | 50 | 40 | 30 | 20 | 10 | 0 | −10 | −20 | −30 | −40 | −50 | −60 |
| 5 | 48 | 37 | 27 | 16 | 6 | −5 | −15 | −26 | −36 | −47 | −57 | −68 |
| 10 | 40 | 28 | 16 | 4 | −9 | −21 | −33 | −46 | −58 | −70 | −83 | −95 |
| 15 | 36 | 22 | 9 | −5 | −18 | −36 | −45 | −58 | −72 | −85 | −99 | −112 |
| 20 | 32 | 18 | 4 | −10 | −25 | −39 | −53 | −67 | −82 | −96 | −110 | −124 |
| 25 | 30 | 16 | 0 | −15 | −29 | −44 | −59 | −74 | −88 | −104 | −118 | −133 |
| 30 | 28 | 13 | −2 | −18 | −33 | −48 | −63 | −79 | −94 | −109 | −125 | −140 |
| 35 | 27 | 11 | −4 | −20 | −35 | −49 | −67 | −82 | −98 | −113 | −129 | −145 |
| 40 | 26 | 10 | −6 | −21 | −37 | −53 | −69 | −85 | −100 | −116 | −132 | −148 |

| (Wind speeds greater than 40 MPH have little additional effect) | Little danger (for properly clothed person) | Increasing danger | Great danger |
|---|---|---|---|
| | | Danger from freezing of exposed flesh | |

*Note.* From *Physiology of Fitness* (p. 191) by B.J. Sharkey, 1984, Champaign, IL: Human Kinetics. Copyright 1984 by Brian J. Sharkey. Reprinted by permission.

## What Effect Does High Altitude Have on Exercise?

If you exercise at high altitude you will find that you do not have to do as much exercise to achieve your THR. There is less oxygen in the blood at high altitude, so the heart has to beat more times to deliver the same amount of oxygen to the muscles. Knowing this, simply use your THR as a guide and cut back on the ordinary intensity of your exercise so that you are able to work out long enough to achieve your caloric expenditure goal. Be sure to take in plenty of fluids, as the dry high-altitude air favors evaporation of sweat from the skin and the respiratory tract.

### What About Exercising in Polluted Air?

Some sections of the country have major pollution problems that can cause you difficulty even when you are at rest. When you exercise under these conditions, these pollutants can irritate the respiratory tract, leading to an asthmatic attack, or they can simply decrease the supply of oxygen in the blood. *Sulfur dioxide* and *ozone* can cause bronchospasms, leading to the wheezing associated with asthma. High temperature and humidity enhance this effect. *Carbon monoxide* is produced by the incomplete combustion of fuels or tobacco and binds to hemoglobin in the blood 200 times more readily than does oxygen. For this reason, even a very small amount of carbon monoxide can decrease oxygen delivery and cause the heart rate to be higher than it would be in an unpolluted environment. In nonsmokers only 1% of the hemoglobin is tied up with carbon monoxide, while the value jumps to 5% for nonsmoking residents of urban areas and 10% for smokers. Performance is affected when the value is at 3%.

## Summary

This chapter provided you with safety tips for exercising in hot, humid, cold, or polluted environments and at high altitude. Heat injury's signs and symptoms can vary from headaches and nausea to extremely high body temperatures that are life-threatening. Prevention is the key; you must focus on exercising in an environment that facilitates the evaporation of sweat and does not impose a large heat load. Wear cotton (or mesh) fabrics that allow the sweat to wick to the surface for evaporation. Gradually increase your exposure to a hot environment so that your body adapts by sweating *more*. Drink water before, during, and after a workout. You should not have to increase your salt intake, as most people take in more than they need with the foods they normally eat. Wear clothing in layers when exercising in the cold and remove the layers to reduce sweating as you warm up. At high altitude use your THR as a guide and reduce exercise intensity to accommodate 30 to 40 minutes of exercise.

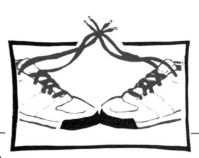

Chapter
*18*

# *Beyond Exercise*

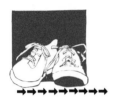

> **Exercise as an End in Itself?**
> **Exercise as a Means to a Better Life?**

This book has tried to give you the information necessary to begin and continue a safe and healthy exercise program. We have assumed that you are interested in fitness in terms of your positive health. This final chapter deals with some subjective observations concerning the direct and indirect value of exercise. We will not examine these ideas in a comprehensive way, but we hope that by sketching the bare outlines of these topics, we will stimulate your imagination so that you can provide the content in ways that are meaningful to you.

## What Does Exercise Bring to My Life?

Exercise can be valuable in our lives simply by virtue of its nature as an activity. Exercise would be good for us even if it had no health benefits. By selecting the type of exercise and the environment in which it is done, exercise can provide for some of our seemingly opposite needs. It can help us whether we need to be

| | | |
|---|---|---|
| learning discipline | or | having fun; |
| serious | or | frivolous; |
| alone with our thoughts | or | enjoying others; |
| using time wisely | or | not using time badly. |

Many regular exercisers know how good it feels to have the discipline to complete a workout even on busy days. At other times, the workout is fun for its own sake as we move in different ways, play games with modified rules, or simply become aware of our natural surroundings while exercising. Exercise can allow for serious contemplation as we plan an upcoming task or a replay of a major life event while we walk or jog. At other times, exercise is done in the most frivolous way as we joke with our exercise companions. Because of the potential benefits of exercise, we are using our time wisely. At the same time, exercise uses time that we might otherwise have used in unhealthy ways (e.g., several hours per week spent eating junk food or smoking).

If you feel the need to achieve some of these qualities but have not yet found them in your fitness program, try exercising in ways that deal with what you think is missing. For example, if you normally exercise with others, try taking a long walk or jog by yourself before an important speech or decision.

Another important aspect of exercise involves what it allows us to do as a result. Exercise provides us with the physical base to more nearly accomplish our goals in other areas of our lives. Increased health and vitality give us enhanced possibilities at home, at work, and in our leisure. The good feeling that often results from exercise helps us approach other parts of our lives with a positive attitude. If you don't experience these results from your exercise program, consider making some modifications in your program to try to achieve these things that many others have found through exercise.

## Finally

One major factor determines whether exercise will bring you its full benefits: *You*. You must decide to include exercise as a regular part of your life. It has to have the same priority status as eating, sleeping, and brushing your teeth. You must find time for exercise almost every day, just as you find time to eat two to three times per day, brush your teeth daily, and sleep at night. You cannot assess such a low priority to exercise that you end up doing it only if you have time left after everything else, only if the weather is nice, only if your friend calls and asks you to play. Your health and physical well-being is worth a few hours per week. Decide that you are going to begin exercise now and continue it for the rest of your life. That is not the only decision you will have to make, but it is one decision that is essential to a quality lifestyle.

## Summary

Exercise has value both for its intrinsic nature and for the benefits that result from doing it on a regular basis. You must decide that it is important enough to include as a vital part of your life *starting now*.

# *Appendixes*

Recommended Dietary Allowances

Estimated Safe and Adequate Dietary Intakes
of Selected Vitamins and Minerals

## Appendix A
### Recommended Daily Dietary Allowances, Revised 1980
Designed for the Maintenance of Good Nutrition of Practically All Healthy People in the U.S.A.

| | Age (years) | Weight (kg) (lbs) | Height (cm) (in) | Protein (g) | Fat-soluble vitamins | | | Water-soluble vitamins | | | | | | | Minerals | | | | | |
|---|---|---|---|---|---|---|---|---|---|---|---|---|---|---|---|---|---|---|---|---|
| | | | | | Vitamin A (µg R.E.)[a] | Vitamin D (µg)[b] | Vitamin E (mg α-T.E.)[c] | Vitamin C (mg) | Thiamin (mg) | Riboflavin (mg) | Niacin (mg N.E.)[d] | Vitamin $B_6$ (mg) | Folacin (µg)[e] | Vitamin $B_{12}$ (µg)[f] | Calcium (mg) | Phosphorus (mg) | Magnesium (mg) | Iron (mg)[g] | Zinc (mg) | Iodine (µg) |
| Infants | 0.0-0.5 | 6 / 13 | 60 / 24 | kg × 2.2 | 420 | 10 | 3 | 35 | 0.3 | 0.4 | 6 | 0.3 | 30 | 0.5[g] | 360 | 240 | 50 | 10 | 3 | 40 |
| | 0.5-1.0 | 9 / 20 | 71 / 28 | kg × 2.0 | 400 | 10 | 4 | 35 | 0.5 | 0.6 | 8 | 0.6 | 45 | 1.5 | 540 | 360 | 70 | 15 | 5 | 50 |
| Children | 1-3 | 13 / 29 | 90 / 35 | 23 | 400 | 10 | 5 | 45 | 0.7 | 0.8 | 9 | 0.9 | 100 | 2.0 | 800 | 800 | 150 | 15 | 10 | 70 |
| | 4-6 | 20 / 44 | 112 / 44 | 30 | 500 | 10 | 6 | 45 | 0.9 | 1.0 | 11 | 1.3 | 200 | 2.5 | 800 | 800 | 200 | 10 | 10 | 90 |
| | 7-10 | 28 / 62 | 132 / 52 | 34 | 700 | 10 | 7 | 45 | 1.2 | 1.4 | 16 | 1.6 | 300 | 3.0 | 800 | 800 | 250 | 10 | 10 | 120 |
| Males | 11-14 | 45 / 99 | 157 / 62 | 45 | 1000 | 10 | 8 | 50 | 1.4 | 1.6 | 18 | 1.8 | 400 | 3.0 | 1200 | 1200 | 350 | 18 | 15 | 150 |
| | 15-18 | 66 / 145 | 176 / 69 | 56 | 1000 | 10 | 10 | 60 | 1.4 | 1.7 | 18 | 2.0 | 400 | 3.0 | 1200 | 1200 | 400 | 18 | 15 | 150 |
| | 19-22 | 70 / 154 | 177 / 70 | 56 | 1000 | 7.5 | 10 | 60 | 1.5 | 1.7 | 19 | 2.2 | 400 | 3.0 | 800 | 800 | 350 | 10 | 15 | 150 |
| | 23-50 | 70 / 154 | 178 / 70 | 56 | 1000 | 5 | 10 | 60 | 1.4 | 1.6 | 18 | 2.2 | 400 | 3.0 | 800 | 800 | 350 | 10 | 15 | 150 |
| | 51+ | 70 / 154 | 178 / 70 | 56 | 1000 | 5 | 10 | 60 | 1.2 | 1.4 | 16 | 2.2 | 400 | 3.0 | 800 | 800 | 350 | 10 | 15 | 150 |

| | | | | | | | | | | | | | | | | | | | | | |
|---|---|---|---|---|---|---|---|---|---|---|---|---|---|---|---|---|---|---|---|---|---|
| Females | 11-14 | 46 | 101 | 157 | 62 | 46 | 800 | 10 | 8 | 50 | 1.1 | 1.3 | 15 | 1.8 | 400 | 3.0 | 1200 | 1200 | 300 | 18 | 15 | 150 |
| | 15-18 | 55 | 120 | 163 | 64 | 46 | 800 | 10 | 8 | 60 | 1.1 | 1.3 | 14 | 2.0 | 400 | 3.0 | 1200 | 1200 | 300 | 18 | 15 | 150 |
| | 19-22 | 55 | 120 | 163 | 64 | 44 | 800 | 7.5 | 8 | 60 | 1.1 | 1.3 | 14 | 2.0 | 400 | 3.0 | 800 | 800 | 300 | 18 | 15 | 150 |
| | 23-50 | 55 | 120 | 163 | 64 | 44 | 800 | 5 | 8 | 60 | 1.0 | 1.2 | 13 | 2.0 | 400 | 3.0 | 800 | 800 | 300 | 18 | 15 | 150 |
| | 51+ | 55 | 120 | 163 | 64 | 44 | 800 | 5 | 8 | 60 | 1.0 | 1.2 | 13 | 2.0 | 400 | 3.0 | 800 | 800 | 300 | 10 | 15 | 150 |
| Pregnant | | | | | | +30 | +200 | +5 | +2 | +20 | +0.4 | +0.3 | +2 | +0.6 | +400 | +1.0 | +400 | +400 | +150 | g | +5 | +25 |
| Lactating | | | | | | +20 | +400 | +5 | +3 | +40 | +0.5 | +0.5 | +5 | +0.5 | +100 | +1.0 | +400 | +400 | +150 | g | +10 | +50 |

*Note.* The allowances are intended to provide for individual variations among most normal persons as they live in the United States under usual environmental stresses. Diets should be based on a variety of common foods in order to provide other nutrients for which human requirements have been less well defined. Reprinted from "Recommended Dietary Allowances," ninth revised edition, 1980, with permission of the National Academy Press, Washington, DC.

[a] Retinol equivalents. 1 Retinol equivalent = 1 µg retinol or 6 µg β carotene.

[b] As cholecalciferol. 10 µg cholecalciferol = 400 I.U. vitamin D.

[c] α-tocopherol equivalents. 1 mg d-α-tocopherol = 1 α T.E.

[d] 1 N.E. (niacin equivalent) is equal to 1 mg of niacin or 60 mg of dietary tryptophan.

[e] The folacin allowances refer to dietary sources as determined by *Lactobacillus casei* assay after treatment with enzymes (conjugases) to make polyglutamyl forms of the vitamin available to the test organism.

[f] The RDA for vitamin $B_{12}$ in infants is based on average concentration of the vitamin in human milk. The allowances after weaning are based on energy intake (as recommended by the American Academy of Pediatrics) and consideration of other factors such as intestinal absorption.

[g] The increased requirement during pregnancy cannot be met by the iron content of habitual American diets nor by the existing iron stores of many women; therefore the use of 30-60 mg of supplemental iron is recommended. Iron needs during lactation are not substantially different from those of nonpregnant women, but continued supplementation of the mother for 2-3 months after parturition is advisable in order to replenish stores depleted by pregnancy.

## Appendix B
### Estimated Safe and Adequate Daily Dietary Intakes of Selected Vitamins and Minerals

| | Age (years) | Vitamins | | | Trace elements[a] | | | | | | Electrolytes | | |
|---|---|---|---|---|---|---|---|---|---|---|---|---|---|
| | | Vitamin K (μg) | Biotin (μg) | Pantothenic acid (mg) | Copper (mg) | Manganese (mg) | Fluoride (mg) | Chromium (mg) | Selenium (mg) | Molybdenum (mg) | Sodium (mg) | Potassium (mg) | Chloride (mg) |
| Infants | 0-0.5 | 12 | 35 | 2 | 0.5-0.7 | 0.5-0.7 | 0.1-0.5 | 0.01-0.04 | 0.01-0.04 | 0.03-0.06 | 115-350 | 350-925 | 275-700 |
| | 0.5-1 | 10-20 | 50 | 3 | 0.7-1.0 | 0.7-1.0 | 0.2-1.0 | 0.02-0.06 | 0.02-0.06 | 0.04-0.08 | 250-750 | 425-1275 | 400-1200 |
| Children | 1-3 | 15-30 | 65 | 3 | 1.0-1.5 | 1.0-1.5 | 0.5-1.5 | 0.02-0.08 | 0.02-0.08 | 0.05-0.1 | 325-975 | 550-1650 | 500-1500 |
| and | 4-6 | 20-40 | 85 | 3-4 | 1.5-2.0 | 1.5-2.0 | 1.0-2.5 | 0.03-0.12 | 0.03-0.12 | 0.06-0.15 | 450-1350 | 775-2325 | 700-2100 |
| adolescents | 7-10 | 30-60 | 120 | 4-5 | 2.0-2.5 | 2.0-3.0 | 1.5-2.5 | 0.05-0.2 | 0.05-0.2 | 0.1 -0.3 | 600-1800 | 1000-3000 | 925-2775 |
| | 11+ | 50-100 | 100-200 | 4-7 | 2.0-3.0 | 2.5-5.0 | 1.5-2.5 | 0.05-0.2 | 0.05-0.2 | 0.15-0.5 | 900-2700 | 1525-4575 | 1400-4200 |
| Adults | | 70-140 | 100-200 | 4-7 | 2.0-3.0 | 2.5-5.0 | 1.5-4.0 | 0.05-0.2 | 0.05-0.2 | 0.15-0.5 | 1100-3300 | 1875-5625 | 1700-5100 |

*Note.* Reprinted from "Recommended Dietary Allowances," ninth revised edition, 1980, with permission of the National Academy Press, Washington, DC. Because there is less information on which to base allowances, these figures are not given in the main table of the RDA and are provided here in the form of ranges of recommended intake.

[a]Because the toxic levels for many trace elements may be only several times usual intakes, the upper levels for the trace elements given in this table should not be habitually exceeded.

# Glossary

The following list of words are terms with which the fitness participant will come into contact. The meanings are related to physical fitness. Many of these words have more general and/or alternative meanings. The health and fitness implications of appropriate terms are noted.

**Abdominal muscular endurance**—the ability of the muscles in the abdominal area to continue to contract without fatigue. Abdominal muscular endurance appears to be an important element in the prevention of low-back pain.

**Acclimatization**—a physiological adaptation to a new environment. For example, a person can do the same work with less effort and can do more total work after becoming acclimatized to a higher altitude (or temperature).

**Active**—communicating motion, as opposed to being passive. Active people include regular physical activity as a part of their lifestyles.

**Adaptation**—the ability to adjust mentally and physically to circumstances or a changing situation. Acclimatization is one example of adaptation.

**Adherence**—state of continuing. Often used to describe people who continue to participate in a physical fitness program.

**Adipose tissue**—a connective tissue in which fat is stored.

**Aerobic activities**—the activities of moderate intensity that use large muscle groups with energy supplied aerobically.

**Aerobic activities**—the activities of moderate intensity that use large muscle groups with energy supplied by processes requiring oxygen.

**Altitude**—the height above sea level for a given point. A person has lower maximal aerobic power with increasing altitudes because of the decreased partial pressure of oxygen in the air.

**Anaerobic threshold**—the point where the metabolic demands of exercise cannot be met aerobically.

**Angina, angina pectoris**—severe cardiac pain which may radiate to the jaws, arms, or legs.

**Anorexia**—an abnormal lack of appetite.

**Apparently healthy**—a term used to describe people without a known disease or illness. These people may vary widely in terms of levels of physical fitness (or positive health).

**Aquatics**—physical activities performed on or in water.

**Arteriosclerosis**—an arterial disease characterized by the hardening and thickening of vessel walls.

**Atherosclerosis**—a disease in which the inner layer of the artery wall becomes thick and irregular with deposits of fatty substances.

**Athlete's foot**—a foot fungus often accompanied by a bacterial infection that causes itching, redness, and a rash on the soles, toes, or between toes.

**Ballistic movement**—a rapid movement.

**Basal metabolic rate**—the minimum energy expenditure required for life in the resting, postabsorptive state.

**Blood pressure**—the pressure exerted by the blood on the vessel walls, measured in millimeters of mercury by the sphygmomanometer. The systolic pressure (SBP, when the left ventricle is in maximal contraction) is the first sound, followed by the diastolic pressure (DBP, when the left ventricle is at rest) which is recorded when there is a change of tone of the sound.

**Body composition**—the relative amounts of muscle, bone, and fat in the body. Body composition is usually divided into fatness (% body fat) and lean body mass (% lean body mass).

**Calisthenics**—exercise without equipment performed for flexibility or muscular development.

**Caloric cost**—the number of calories used for a specific task, normally reported in kcal/min.

**Calorie**—calorie = .001 kilocalories = amount of heat required to raise the temperature of 1 g of water 1 °C.

**Carbohydrate**—dietary nutrient including sugars, cellulose, and starches.

**Cardiac output**—the amount of blood circulated by the heart each minute; cardiac output = heart rate × stroke volume.

**Cardiac rehabilitation**—a program designed to help cardiac patients return to normal lives with reduced risk of additional health problems.

**Cardiopulmonary resuscitation (CPR)**—a method to restore normal pulse and breathing by mouth-to-mouth respiration and rhythmical compression on the chest. People working in fitness programs should be certified in CPR.

**Cardiorespiratory function**—pertaining to the heart and respiration.

**Cardiovascular**—pertaining to the heart and blood vessels.

**Cellulite**—a label given to lumpy deposits of fat commonly appearing on the back and front of the legs and buttocks in overweight individuals.

**Cholesterol**—a fat-like substance found in animal tissues. The healthy plasma level is considered to be below 200 milligrams per 100 milliliters. Higher levels are associated with increased risk of atherosclerosis.

**Circuit training**—a sequence of exercises done one after the other in the same workout.

**Competitive running**—running in a race with the main objective of trying to win the race.

**Concentric contraction**—a shortening of the muscle as a result of the contraction of that muscle.

**Conditioning**—chronic physical training.

**Contraindications**—a sign or symptom suggesting that a certain activity should be avoided.

**Cool-down; taper-down**—a period of light activity following moderate to heavy exercise. The cool-down period is important because the leg muscles continue to pump blood back to the heart, whereas stopping immediately after exercise causes pooling of the blood in the legs and a lack of venous return.

**Coronary-prone personality**—a person with "Type A" behavior (e.g., hard-driving, impatient, time-conscious). Someone with a coronary-prone personality may have a higher risk of CHD.

**Cross adaptation**—the transfer of increased adaptation from one stimulus (or stressor) to another stimulus. For example, some have claimed that increased adaptation to physical work from physical conditioning carries over to better adaptation to mental or emotional stressors. The evidence is not clear.

**Cycle ergometer**—a one-wheeled stationary cycle with adjustable resistance used as a work task for exercise testing or conditioning.

**Dehydration**—the excessive loss of body fluids.

**Detrained**—the results of becoming sedentary after a physical conditioning program. The effects (e.g., increased fat, decreased CRF) are opposite those of conditioning.

**Diabetes**—a metabolic disorder characterized by an inability to oxidize carbohydrates because of the disturbance of the normal insulin mechanism.

**Diastolic blood pressure (DBP)**—the pressure exerted by the blood on the vessel walls, measured in millimeters of mercury by a sphygmomanometer, when the left ventricle is at rest.

**Diet**—the food eaten by an individual. Diet sometimes refers to a special selection of food.

**Duration**—length of time for a fitness workout. Guidelines often include 15-30 min of aerobic work at a target heart rate; however, more importantly, the total work accomplished (e.g., distance covered) should be emphasized.

**Eccentric contraction**—a lengthening of the muscle during its contraction.

**Emotion**—a strong feeling, often accomplished by stress reactions and behaviors.

**End point**—the point at which an exercise test is changed to the taper down or stopped.

**Endurance run**—a race of a set distance (for time) or set time (for distance). Normally used to determine a person's cardiorespiratory endurance. Runs of at least 1 mile or 6 min should be used.

**Energy**—the capacity for performing work, often measured in terms of oxygen consumption.

**Evaluation**—the determination or judgment of the value or worth of something or someone. In a fitness setting, an evaluation determines the health or fitness status of an individual based on his or her characteristics, signs, symptoms, behaviors, and test results.

**Evaporation**—conversion from the liquid to the gaseous state by means of heat, as in evaporation of sweat.

**Exercise**—physical activity, normally of large muscle groups, in a continuous manner, at a certain intensity and frequency, resulting in enough total work so that desirable fitness changes are made and maintained.

**Exercise components**—warm-up, main body of exercise, and taper-down.

**Exercise modification**—adjustment to a person's exercise program in terms of type of activity, intensity, frequency, and/or total work accomplished to more nearly achieve the fitness goals.

**Exercise prescription**—a recommendation for a fitness program in terms of type of activities, intensity, frequency, and total amount of work aimed at producing or maintaining desirable fitness objectives.

**Exercise progression**—the increase in total work and/or intensity as a person gradually goes from a sedentary lifestyle to the recommended levels of physical activity.

**Extension**—increasing the angle at a joint, such as straightening the elbow.

**Extrinsic**—external, as in extrinsic motivation (e.g., reward) to begin or continue exercise.

**Family history**—refers to the major health problems that have been found in a person's grandparents, parents, uncles/aunts, and siblings. Heart disease in a person's family is a secondary risk factor for CHD.

**Fat**—a compound containing glycerol and fatty acids which is used as a source of energy and can be stored in the body.

**Fat-free weight**, also **lean body weight**—the amount of total body weight that is free of fat; equal to total body weight minus fat weight.

**Fat weight**—the absolute amount of total body weight that is body fat; equal to total body weight times percent fat.

**Field tests**—tests that can be used in mass testing situations.

**Fitness**—a state of health characteristics, symptoms, and behaviors enabling a person to have the highest quality of life. Increases in fitness components are related to positive health, whereas decreases in fitness components increase the risk of major health problems.

**Fitness activities**—actions that lead to increased fitness.

**Fitness center**—an organization that provides fitness tests, activities, and evaluations.

**Fitness instructor**—a person who assists people in evaluating and improving fitness. Certification is offered by the American College of Sports Medicine for health/fitness instructors who work with apparently healthy populations.

**Fitness program**—an organized series of activities aimed at promoting increased fitness.

**Fitness testing**—the measurement and evaluation of status of all fitness components.

**Fitness workout**—a specific fitness session.

**Flexibility**—the ability to move a joint through the full range of motion without discomfort or pain.

**Frequency**—how often a person has a fitness workout (usually days per week).

**Fun run**—a race with an emphasis on participation (as opposed to winning).

**Functional capacity**—maximal oxygen uptake, expressed in milliliters of oxygen per kilogram of body weight per minute, or in METs.

**Games**—a form of playing for amusement. Games may be cooperative or competitive, involving a few or many people. Games can also be used to achieve fitness improvements.

**Genetic potential**—the possibilities and limits imposed by a person's inherited genes.

**Graded Exercise Test (GXT)**—a multistage test that determines a person's physiological response to different intensities of exercise and/or the person's peak aerobic power.

**Gram (g)**—a basic unit of mass in the metric system. 1,000 g = 1 kg.

**Health**—the absence of disease is the minimum level. Positive health includes the ability of a person to pursue his or her goals.

**Health history**—information about a person's past health record.

**Health-related attitudes**—a manner of thinking associated with healthy behaviors.

**Health-related behavior**—a person's actions that are associated with positive or negative health.

**Health-related sign**—evidence of something with a potential health consequence.

**Health-related symptom**—a sensation that arises from or accompanies a particular disease or disorder and serves as an indicator of it.

**Health status**—the current level of disease and fitness.

**Healthy life**—a lifestyle including behaviors related to enhanced fitness and excluding harmful behaviors.

**Heart**—the hollow muscular organ that pumps the blood through the body. The heart lies obliquely between the two lungs, behind the sternum. The heart is composed of four chambers, left and right atria, and ventricles.

**Heart attack**—a general term used to describe an acute episode of heart disease.

**Heart disease**—a general term used to describe any of several abnormalities of the heart causing it to be unable to function properly.

**Heart rate**—the number of beats of the heart per minute.

**Heat cramps**—a spasmodic contraction of a muscle or group of muscles which is caused by working in extreme heat.

**Heat exhaustion**—collapse, with or without loss of consciousness, suffered in conditions of heat and high humidity, largely resulting from the loss of fluid and salt by sweating.

**Heat illness**—a general term for problems caused by activity in high temperatures.

**Heat stroke**—the final stage in heat exhaustion. When the body is unable to lose heat, death may ensue.

**Heat syncope**—fainting or sudden loss of strength because of excessive heat gain.

**High blood pressure, hypertension**—blood pressure in excess of normal values.

**High-calorie diet**—food consumption of which the caloric value exceeds the total daily energy requirement, resulting in increased adipose tissue.

**High-density lipoprotein cholesterol (HDL-C)**—a plasma lipid-protein complex containing relatively more protein and less cholesterol and triglycerides. Low levels of HDL-C are associated with CHD.

**Humidity**—the amount of moisture in the atmosphere.

**Hypercholesterolemia**—an excess of cholesterol in the blood.

**Hyperlipemia**—excess fat in the blood.

**Hyperlipoproteinemia**—an increase in the concentration of the three fatty substances of the blood: cholesterol, phospholipid, and triglyceride.

**Hyperplasia**—new fat cell formation.

**Hypertension**—high blood pressure. Normally systolic blood pressure exceeds 140 mmHg or diastolic pressure exceeds 90 mmHg in someone who has hypertension.

**Hypertrophy**—an increase in the size of a muscle, organ, or other body part caused by an enlargement of its constituent cells.

**Hypervitaminosis**—a condition in which the level of a vitamin in the blood or tissues is high enough to cause undesirable effects.

**Hypokinetic disease**—a disease that relates to or is caused by the lack of regular physical activity.

**Hypothermia**—below normal body temperature.

**Increment**—a degree of increase. In a graded exercise test a work increment exists between stages.

**Informed consent**—a procedure used to obtain a person's voluntary permission to participate in a program. Informed consent normally requires a description of the procedures to be used, the potential benefits and risks, and written consent.

**Intensity**—the magnitude of energy required for a particular activity, often referred to in terms of percent of max ($\dot{V}O_2$, HR, or METs).

**Intermittent work**—exercises performed with alternate periods of harder and lighter physical work, or work and rest, rather than continuous work.

**Interval training**—a fitness workout that alternates harder and lighter work.

**Intrinsic**—belonging to a thing by its very nature (e.g., people continue to be active based on intrinsic motivation).

**Isokinetic contraction**—a muscle contraction with controlled speed, allowing maximal force to be applied throughout the range of motion.

**Isometric contraction**—a muscle contraction in which the muscle length is unchanged.

**Isotonic contraction**—a muscle contraction in which the force of the muscle is greater than the resistance resulting from joint movement, with shortening or lengthening of the muscle.

**Jogging**—slow running.

**Joint**—the articulation of two or more bones.

**Kilocalorie (kcal) or Calorie (Cal)**—the amount of heat required to raise the temperature of 1 kg of water 1 °C.

**Kilogram (kg)**—a metric unit of mass; 1 kg = 1,000 g.

**Lean body weight**—the portion of the body that is not fat tissue. Lean body weight is often used to refer to all nonfat weight.

**Life events**—situations that cause stress reactions—they may be enjoyable (e.g., a vacation), or sad (e.g., the death of a loved one).

**Lifestyle**—a person's general pattern of living, including healthy and unhealthy behaviors.

**Limiting factor**—a physiological characteristic that establishes the upper limit of performance (e.g., muscle fiber type, maximal cardiac output, maximal oxygen uptake).

**Lipid**—a fatty substance.

**Lipoprotein**—a complex consisting of lipid and protein molecules bound together. Cholesterol and triglycerides are transported in the bloodstream in the form of lipoproteins.

**Low-back function**—the ability to carry on normal activities without back pain.

**Low-back pain**—strong discomfort in the low-back area, often caused by lack of muscular endurance and flexibility in the mid-trunk region, or improper posture or lifting.

**Low-calorie diet**—food intake of which the caloric value is below the total energy requirement, resulting in a loss of weight.

**Low-density lipoprotein cholesterol (LDL-C)**—a plasma protein containing relatively more cholesterol and triglycerides and less protein. High levels are associated with an increased risk of CHD.

**Lumbar**—pertaining to the low back; five lumbar vertebrae are located just below the thoracic vertebrae and just above the sacrum.

**Maintenance load**—the amount of exercise that enables an individual to maintain his or her present level of fitness.

**Malnutrition**—poor or improper nutrition, usually associated with undernutrition.

**Max $\dot{V}O_2$**—see **maximal oxygen uptake**.

**Maximal**—the highest level possible, such as maximal heart rate or oxygen uptake.

**Maximal heart rate**—the highest heart rate attainable. A person's maximal heart rate can be estimated by subtracting his or her age from 220.

**Maximal oxygen uptake**—the greatest rate of oxygen utilization attainable during heavy work, expressed in liters per minute, or ml/[kg × min].

**Maximal tests**—tests that continue until a person has reached a maximal level (e.g., max $\dot{V}O_2$) or voluntary exhaustion.

**Maximum voluntary ventilation**—the maximal amount of air that can be moved in and out of the lungs. A person is normally tested for 10-15 sec, then the result is reported in liters per minute.

**Medical clearance**—an indication by medical personnel that an individual can safely engage in specified activities.

**Medical history**—a person's previous health problems, signs, and characteristics.

**Medical referral**—a recommendation that a person get medical attention, tests, or an opinion about a characteristic, symptom, or test result to determine if medical treatment is needed, and/or to determine whether it is safe to participate in specified activities.

**Medical supervision**—the presence of qualified medical personnel during a fitness test or workout.

**Metabolic load**—the energy required to complete a task.

**Metabolism**—the process of chemical changes by which energy is provided for the maintenance of life.

**METs**—multiples of resting metabolism (1 MET is about 3.5 ml/[kg × min]).

**Millisecond**—one-thousandth (.001) of a second.

**Motivation**—the incentive(s) that prompts a person to act with a sense of purpose.

**Myocardial infarction (MI)**—death to a section of heart tissue in which the blood supply has been cut off.

**Negative energy balance**—a condition in which less energy is consumed than is expended, resulting in a decrease in body weight.

**Negative health**—the presence of characteristics and behaviors that prevent optimal functional capacity and increase risks of serious health problems.

**Nutrients**—compounds and elements contained in foods and needed by the body.

**Nutrition**—the study of foods and their use in the body.

**Obesity**—the accumulation and storage of excess body fat. Obese people have an increased risk of CHD, diabetes, and hypertension.

**One repetition maximum, 1 RM**—the maximal force that can be exerted in a single contraction by a muscle group.

**Ossification**—the replacement of cartilage by bone.

**Overfat**—an accumulation of more than the desirable amount of fat.

**Overload**—to place greater than usual demands upon some part of the body (e.g., picking up more weight than normal overloads the muscles involved). Chronic overloading leads to increased strength and function.

**Overweight**—a person's weight that is greater than expected for his or her height.

**Oxygen**—a colorless, odorless, gaseous element necessary for life and combustion.

**Oxygen consumption**—see **oxygen uptake**.

**Oxygen cost**—the amount of oxygen used by body tissues during an activity.

**Oxygen requirement**—the rate of oxygen utilization needed for an activity.

**Oxygen uptake**—the rate at which oxygen is utilized during a specific level of an activity.

**Palpation**—examination by touch, as in determining HR by feeling the pulse at the wrist or neck.

**Palpitation**—a rapid forceful beating of the heart of which the person is aware.

**Peak heart rate**—the highest heart rate during a specific activity.

**Percent fat**—the percentage of total body weight that is fat.

**Perceived exertion**—a subjective rating of intensity of a particular task, normally rated on one of the Borg scales for rating perceived exertion.

**Performance**—the carrying out of a task that requires effort, attention, and skill. A person's success depends on his or her ability to perform a specific task.

**Phases of activities**—the sequence of exercise recommended to progress from a sedentary to an active lifestyle, including a gradual progression to walking 4 mi and jogging 3 mi, including a variety of sports and games.

**Physical conditioning**—chronic regular exercise aimed at obtaining or maintaining high levels of components of fitness.

**Physical fitness**—the physical aspects of total well-being related to optimal functional capacity and low risks of serious health problems.

**Physical fitness profile**—a description of the levels of the components of physical fitness.

**Physical fitness tests**—ways to measure and evaluate the components of physical fitness.

**Physical inactivity**—a sedentary lifestyle.

**Physical work capacity**—the capacity to perform physical work, usually measured in oxygen uptake or kilopond meters per minute while at a set heart rate (e.g., PWC-150).

**Physiological response**—the reaction of the physiological systems to a task, condition, or stressor.

**Polyunsaturated fats**—fats derived from vegetables, lean poultry, fish, and cereal.

**Positive energy balance**—a condition in which more energy is consumed than is expended, resulting in an increase in body weight.

**Positive health**—a move toward optimal functioning; more than a mere absence of disease.

**Posture**—the position or carriage of the body as a whole. Improper posture is related to low-back pain.

**Predicted maximum heart rate**—an estimate of max HR; 220 minus a person's age.

**Prescribed exercise**—a recommendation of type, intensity, frequency, duration, and total work needed to accomplish fitness objectives.

**Primary risk factor**—a characteristic or behavior that is associated with a major health problem regardless of other factors. For example, smoking is a primary risk factor of CHD.

**Progression**—a gradual increase from a current level to a desired level. For example, a sedentary person may gradually increase walking and jogging until he or she is able to jog 3 mi continuously without discomfort over an 8-month period of time.

**Protein**—a compound composed of amino acids that provides the basic structural properties of cells.

**Psychological stressor**—a mental condition that causes physiological arousal beyond what is needed to accomplish a task.

**Pulmonary**—pertaining to the lungs.

**Pulmonary function**—the capacity of the lungs. Pulmonary function is often tested by measuring vital capacity, maximal expiratory force, and maximal voluntary ventilation.

**Radial pulse**—a pulse taken at the wrist.

**Rating of perceived exertion**—a scale, by Borg, used to quantify the subjective feeling of physical effort. The original scale was 6-20; the revised scale is 0-10.

**Recommended Dietary Allowance (RDA)**—the quantities of daily specified vitamins, minerals, and proteins needed for good nutrition.

**Relax**—to loosen, make less stiff, or gain relief from work or tension.

**Repetitions**—the number of consecutive contractions performed.

**Resistance**—the amount of force applied opposite a movement.

**Respiration**—the act or function of breathing.

**Risk factor**—a characteristic, sign, symptom, or test score that is associated with increased probability of developing a health problem. For example, people with hypertension have an increased risk of developing CHD.

**Running**—moving the whole body quickly by propelling the body off the ground during part of the movement.

**Running shoes**—special athletic shoes offering good support and cushioning in the heel area to minimize trauma at impact.

**Saturated fat**—a fat that is not capable of absorbing any more hydrogen. These fats are solid at room temperature and are usually of animal origin such as the fats in milk, butter, and meat.

**Screening**—an examination used to select or reject. In fitness programs, potential participants are screened to determine whether they should be referred for medical attention prior to engaging in exercise.

**Secondary risk factor**—a characteristic, sign, symptom, or test score that has a weak independent association with a health problem, but increases the risk when other risk factors are present.

**Sedentary**—an inactive lifestyle, characterized by a lot of sitting.

**Sequence of testing**—the logical order in which tests are conducted.

**Set**—a designated number of repetitions.

**Skinfold caliper**—an instrument used to measure the thickness of folds of fat that have been pinched away from the body.

**Specificity**—belonging to and characteristic of a particular thing. For example, skill is specific to a certain aspect of a sport.

**Spot reducing**—refers to an effort to reduce fat at one site by doing calisthenics at that site. No research evidence supports this concept.

**Stage**—in exercise testing, refers to the step in the levels of work going from light to hard.

**Steady state**—unchanging, or changing very little. For example, during submaximal exercise, a person reaches a steady state (a leveling-off of oxygen, HR, etc.) after a few minutes.

**Strength**—the amount of force that can be exerted by a muscle group against a resistance.

**Stress**—a physiological or psychological response to a stressor beyond what is needed to accomplish a task.

**Stretching**—extending the limbs through a full range of motion.

**Stroke, apoplexy**—the sudden loss of consciousness resulting from a vascular accident in the brain, usually resulting in partial paralysis.

**Stroke volume**—the amount of blood pumped from the left ventricle each time the heart contracts.

**Submaximal**—less than maximal (e.g., an exercise that can be performed with less than maximal effort).

**Supervised fitness program**—a group of fitness activities with an instructor present.

**Symptom**—a noticeable change in the normal working of the body that indicates or accompanies disease or sickness.

**Systolic blood pressure**—the pressure exerted on the vessel walls during ventricular contraction, measured in millimeters of mercury by the sphygmomanometer.

**Taper-down; cool-down**—light activity after a workout, allowing a gradual return to normal, with leg muscles continuing to pump blood back to the heart thus preventing pooling of blood in the lower extremities.

**Target heart rate (THR)**—the heart rate recommended for fitness workouts.

**Testing protocol**—a particular testing scheme, often the starting level, timing, and increments for each stage of an exercise tolerance test.

**Threshold**—the minimum level needed for desired effect. Often used to refer to the minimum level of exercise intensity needed for improvement in cardiorespiratory function.

**Time to exhaustion**—the time interval from the beginning of an exercise test until the participant is unable or unwilling to continue.

**Total work**—the amount of work accomplished during a workout.

**Training**—physical conditioning through repeated bouts of exercise.

**Treadmill**—a machine with a moving belt that can be adjusted for speed and grade allowing a person to walk/run in one place. Treadmills are widely used for exercise tolerance testing.

**Triglyceride**—a compound consisting of three molecules of fatty acid and glycerol. Triglyceride is the main type of lipid found in adipose tissue and the main dietary lipid. When hydrolyzed, triglyceride releases free fatty acids into the bloodstream. A high level of triglyceride in serum is a secondary risk factor of CHD.

**12-minute run**—a field test for cardiorespiratory endurance, scored by the distance run in 12 min.

**2-mile run**—a field test for cardiorespiratory endurance, scored by the time it takes to complete 2 mi.

**Type A behavior**—the characterization of a person who is hard-driving, time conscious, and impatient. Some evidence suggests that this type of behavior is a secondary risk factor of CHD. Type A is the opposite of Type B.

**Type B behavior**—the opposite of Type A behavior.

**Unsaturated fat**—the molecules of a fat, which have one or more double bonds, and are thus capable of absorbing more hydrogen. These fats are liquid at room temperature and usually are of vegetable origin.

**Unsupervised program**—a group of fitness activities without supervision by qualified fitness personnel for people with a low risk of health problems.

**$\dot{V}O_2$max**—the highest amount of oxygen that can be utilized by the body during hard work.

**Ventilation**—the process of oxygenating the blood through the lungs.

**Ventilatory threshold**—the intensity of work at which the rate of ventilation sharply increases.

**Vitamins**—an organic substance that is present in small amounts of food and that is necessary for the normal functioning of the cells. Vitamins are classified as water-soluble (B complex and C) or fat-soluble (A, D, E, K).

**Walking**—moving the body in a set direction while maintaining contact with the ground (floor).

**Warm-up**—physical activity of light to moderate intensity prior to a workout.

**Windchill**—the coldness felt on exposed human flesh by a combination of temperature and wind velocity.

**Work**—movement of a force through a distance; measured as foot-pound, and kilogram, as on a cycle ergometer.

**Workrate**—work done per unit of time (e.g., kilogram meters per minute; watts).

**Work/relief**—the ratio of time spent in more intense and less intense exercise in an interval type of workout.

**Workout**—an exercise bout aimed at improving fitness or performance.

# Bibliography

Althoff, S.A., Svoboda, M., and Girdano, D.A. (1988). *Choices in health and fitness for life*. Scottsdale, AZ: Gorsuch Scarisbrick.

American Alliance for Health, Physical Education, Recreation and Dance. (1980). *Health related physical fitness test manual*. Reston, VA: Author.

American College of Obstetricians and Gynecologists. (1985). *Exercise during pregnancy and the postnatal period (ACOG Home Exercise Programs)*. Washington, DC: Author.

American College of Sports Medicine. (1975). Prevention of heat injuries during distance running. *Medicine and Science in Sports*, **7**, vii-viii.

American College of Sports Medicine. (1978). The recommended quantity and quality of exercise for developing and maintaining fitness in healthy adults. *Medicine and Science in Sports*, **10**, vii-x.

American College of Sports Medicine. (1980). *Guidelines for graded exercise testing and exercise prescription*. Philadelphia: Lea and Febiger.

American College of Sports Medicine. (1983). Proper and improper weight loss programs. *Medicine and Science in Sports and Exercise*, **15**, ix-xiii.

American Diabetic Association & American Dietetic Association. (1986). *Exchange lists* (p. 5). Alexandria, VA, & Chicago, IL: Authors.

American Heart Association. (1978). *Diet and coronary heart disease*. Dallas: Author.

American Heart Association. (1981). *Student manual for basic life support—cardiopulmonary resuscitation*. Dallas: Author.

American Heart Association Committee on Stress, Strain, and Heart Disease. Report. (1977). *Circulation*, **55**, 1-11.

American Red Cross. (1981). *Advanced first aid and emergency care* (2nd ed.). New York: Doubleday.

Anderson, B. (1980). *Stretching*. Bolinas, CA: Shelter.

Blair, S.N., Jacobs, D.R., & Powell, K.E. (1985). Relationships between exercise or physical activity and other health behaviors. *Public Health Reports*, **100**, 180-188.

Blair, S.N., Painter, P., Pate, R.R., Smith, L.K., & Taylor, C.B. (Eds.) (1988). *Resource Manual for Exercise Testing and Prescription*. Philadelphia: Lea & Febiger.

Borg, G.A.V. (1982). Psychological bases of physical exertion. *Medicine and Science in Sports and Exercise*, **14**(5), 377-381.

Bubb, W.J. (1986). Relative leanness. In E.T. Howley & B.D. Franks, *Health/fitness instructor's handbook* (pp. 51-79). Champaign, IL: Human Kinetics.

Carver, S. (1986). Injury prevention and treatment. In E.T. Howley & B.D. Franks, *Health/fitness instructor's handbook* (pp. 211-232). Champaign, IL: Human Kinetics.

Christian, J.L., & Greger, J.L. (1985). *Nutrition for living*. Menlo Park, CA: Benjamin/Cummings.

Cooper, K.H. (1977). *The aerobics way*. New York: Bantam.

Cooper, P.G. (1985). *Aerobics theory and practice.* Sherman Oaks, CA: Aerobics and Fitness Association of America.

Corbin, C.B., & Lindsey, R. (1988). *Concepts of physical fitness* (6th ed.). Dubuque, IA: Wm. C. Brown.

Cureton, T.K. (1965). *Physical fitness and dynamic health.* New York: Dial Press.

Dusek, D.E. (1982). *Thin and fit: Your personal lifestyle.* Belmont, CA: Wadsworth.

Food and Nutrition Board, National Academy of Science—National Research Council. (1980). *Recommended dietary allowances* (9th ed.). Washington, DC: National Academy Press.

Fox, E.L., Kirby, T.E., & Fox, A.R. (1987). *Bases of fitness.* New York: Macmillan.

Getchell, B. (1983). *Physical fitness—a way of life.* (3rd Ed.). New York: Wiley.

Golding, L.A., Myers, C.R., & Sinning, W.E. (Eds.). (1982). *The Y's way to physical fitness.* Chicago: National Board of YMCA.

Hamilton, E.M.N., & Whitney, E.N. (1982). *Nutrition* (2nd Ed.). St. Paul, MN: West.

Hector, M.A. (1986). Behavior modification. In E.T. Howley & B.D. Franks, *Health/fitness instructor's handbook* (pp. 199-207). Champaign, IL: Human Kinetics.

Heyward, V.H. (1984). *Designs for fitness.* Minneapolis: Burgess.

Hockey, R.V. (1985). *Physical fitness: The pathway to healthful living* (5th ed.). St. Louis: Times Mirror/Mosby College.

Holmer, I. (1980). Physiology of swimming man. *Exercise and Sport Sciences Reviews,* **7**, pp. 87-123.

Howley, E.T., & Franks, B.D. (1986). *Health/fitness instructor's handbook.* Champaign, IL: Human Kinetics.

Jackson, A.S., & Pollock, M.L. (1985). Practical assessment of body composition. *The Physician and Sportsmedicine,* **13**, 76-90.

Kasch, F.W. (1976). The effects of exercise on the aging process. *The Physician and Sportsmedicine,* **4**(6), 64-68.

Katch, F.I., & McArdle, W.D. (1977). *Nutrition, weight control, and exercise.* Boston: Houghton Mifflin.

Kline, G.M., Porcari, J.P., Hintermeister, R., Freedson, P.S., Ward, A., McCarron, R.F., Ross, J., & Rippe, J.M. (1987). Estimation of $\dot{V}O_2max$ from a one-mile track walk, gender, age, and body weight. *Medicine and Science in Sports and Exercise,* **19**, 253-259.

Kraus, H., & Raab, W. (1961). *Hypokinetic disease.* Springfield, IL: Charles C Thomas.

Lewis, J.L. (1986). Anatomy and kinesiology. In E.T. Howley & B.D. Franks, *Health/fitness instructor's handbook* (pp. 37-48). Champaign, IL: Human Kinetics.

Lohman, T.G. (November/December, 1987). The use of skinfolds to estimate body fatness in children and youth. *Journal of Physical Education, Recreation and Dance,* **58**, 98-102.

Martin, A.D. (1986). ECG and medications. In E.T. Howley & B.D. Franks, *Health/fitness instructor's handbook* (pp. 185-198). Champaign, IL: Human Kinetics.

McArdle, W.D., Katch, F.I., and Katch, V.L. (1981). *Exercise Physiology.* Philadelphia: Lea and Febiger.

Melleby, A. (1982). *The Y's way to a healthy back.* Piscataway, NJ: New Century.

Metropolitan Life Insurance Company of New York. (1959). New weight standards for men and women. *Statistical Bulletin*, **40**, 1-4.

Miller, D.K., & Allen, T.E. (1986). *Fitness: A lifetime commitment* (3rd ed.). Edina, MN: Burgess.

Montoye, H.J. (1975). *Physical activity and health: An epidemiologic study of an entire community*. Englewood Cliffs: Prentice-Hall.

Morgan, W.P. (1985). Affective beneficence of vigorous physical activity. *Medicine and Science in Sports and Exercise*, **17**, 94-100.

National Research Council & National Academy of Sciences. (1980). *Recommended dietary allowances* (p. 178 and foldout). Washington, DC: National Academy Press.

National Institute on Alcohol Abuse and Alcoholism. (1971, 1974, & 1978). *Alcohol and health* (Reports to the U.S. Congress). Washington, DC: U.S. Government Printing Office.

New Games Foundation (1976). *The new games book*. Garden City, NY: Dolphin.

Nieman, D.C. (1985). *Health related physical fitness*. Loma Linda, CA: School of Health, Loma Linda University.

Paffenbarger, R.S., & Hyde, R.T. (1984). Exercise in the prevention of coronary heart disease. *Preventive Medicine*, **13**, 3-22.

Paffenbarger, R.S., Wing, A.L., Hyde, R.T., & Jung, D.L. (1983). Physical activity and incidence of hypertension in college alumni. *American Journal of Epidemiology*, **117**, 245-256.

Pollock, M.L., Wilmore, J.H., & Fox, S.M. (1984). *Exercise in health and disease*. Philadelphia: W.B. Saunders.

Seefeldt, V., & Vogel, P. (1986). *The value of physical activity*. Reston, VA: American Alliance for Health, Physical Education, Recreation and Dance.

Selye, H. (1956). *Stress of life*. New York: McGraw-Hill.

Selye, H. (1974). *Stress without distress*. Toronto: McCelland & Stewart.

Selye, H. (1976). Stress and physical activity. *McGill Journal of Education*, **11**, 3-14.

Sharkey, B.J. (1984). *Physiology of fitness*. Champaign, IL: Human Kinetics.

Sharpe, G.S., & Liemohn, W.P. (1986). Strength, endurance, and flexibility. In E.T. Howley and B.D. Franks, *Health/fitness instructor's handbook* (pp. 99-113). Champaign, IL.: Human Kinetics.

Smith, E.L., & Gilligan, C. (1987). Effects of inactivity and exercise on bone. *The Physician and Sportsmedicine*, **15**(11), 91-102.

Stuart, R.B., and Davies, B. (1971). *Slim chance in a fat world: Behavioral control of obesity*. Champaign, IL: Research Press.

U.S. Department of Health & Human Services. (1980). *Promoting health/ preventing disease: Objectives for the nation*. Washington, DC: U.S. Government Printing Office.

U.S. Department of Health & Human Services. (1981). *Exercise and your heart*. Washington, DC: U.S. Government Printing Office.

U.S. Department of Health & Human Services, Public Health Service, Office on Smoking and Health. (1983). *The health consequences of smoking: Cardiovascular disease, a report of the Surgeon General* (DHEW Publication No. PHS 79-50066). Washington, DC: U.S. Government Printing Office.

U.S. Senate Select Committee on Nutrition and Human Needs. (1977). Dietary Goals for the United States (Stock No. 052 070 043 768). Washington, DC: U.S. Government Printing Office.

Williams, M.H. (1988). *Nutrition for fitness and sport* (2nd ed.). Dubuque, IA: Wm. C. Brown.

Williams, P.C. (1974). *Low back and neck pain*. Springfield, IL: Charles C Thomas.

Williams, R.L., & Long, J.D. (1983). *Toward a self-managed life style*. Boston: Houghton Mifflin.

Wilmore, J.H. (1986). *Sensible fitness*. Champaign, IL: Human Kinetics.

Wilmoth, S.K. (1986). *Leading aerobic dance-exercise*. Champaign, IL: Human Kinetics.

World Health Organization. (1982). *Prevention of coronary heart disease*. Geneva: Author.

# Index

# About the Authors and Illustrators

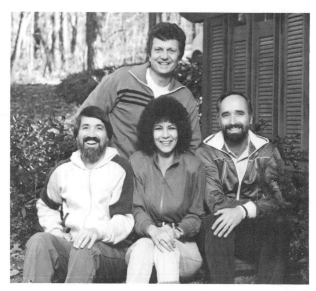

**Front,** (*left to right*): Don Franks, Susan Metros, and Ed Howley
**Back**: George Moudry

**B. Don Franks** grew up in Arkansas and received his BS and MEd degrees in physical education from the University of Arkansas, Fayetteville. He received his PhD in physical education from the University of Illinois at Urbana-Champaign. Dr. Franks is a professor and the director of the School of Health, Physical Education, Recreation, and Dance at Louisiana State University, Baton Rouge. His research interest is the cardiovascular response to exercise and psychological stressors.

Dr. Franks is a Fellow of the American Academy of Physical Education, the American College of Sports Medicine, and the Research Consortium of the American Alliance for Health, Physical Education, Recreation and Dance. He has served as president of the AAHPERD Research Consortium, advocating a "health-related" approach to physical fitness.

In his spare time, Dr. Franks enjoys playing basketball, badminton, and racquetball as well as reading novels and attending jazz and drama performances.

**Edward T. Howley** received his PhD in physical education from the University of Wisconsin, Madison. He is a professor and the director of the Applied Physiology Research Laboratory at the University of Tennessee, Knoxville, where he received the Alumni Association Outstanding Teaching Award. His research interests include the measurement of the metabolic costs of physical activities and the evaluation of hormonal responses to exercise and other stressors.

Dr. Howley has been active as a Fellow in the American College of Sports Medicine and as president of its Southeast Chapter. He also served on the ACSM Preventive and Rehabilitative Committee that developed the college's various certification programs.

In his leisure time, Dr. Howley enjoys paddleball, soccer, and golf.

In addition to *Fitness Leader's Handbook* and *Fitness Facts*, Don Franks and Ed Howley coauthored *Health/Fitness Instructor's Handbook*.

**Susan E. Metros**, who designed the introductory symbols used in the book, received her BS in painting and drawing and her MS in graphic design from Michigan State University. She is an associate professor of art and the director of the Computer-Enhanced Design Laboratory at the University of Tennessee, Knoxville. As an educator, she has developed, prepared, and taught courses in design production and processing. Professor Metros is a consultant to education, industry, business, and government concerning issues related to graphic design, creative problem solving, and computer-enhanced design. She has won numerous design awards and is the author of *Design-On-Line: Computer-Enhanced Graphic Design*.

**George Moudry,** the cartoonist, earned his PhD in exercise physiology from the University of Tennessee. He is the director of wellness at St. John Medical Center in Tulsa, Oklahoma. A 10-year veteran of the fitness business, Dr. Moudry has established and operated fitness, wellness, and rehabilitation programs in a variety of settings, including academic, clinical, corporate, and commercial. He is a long-standing member of the Association for Fitness in Business and the American College of Sports Medicine.